2nd edition

review for
USMLE

**United States
Medical Licensing
Examination**

Step 1

2nd edition

review for
USMLE

**United States
Medical Licensing
Examination**

Step **1**

John S. Lazo, Ph.D.

*Chairman, Department of Pharmacology
Allegheny Foundation Professor of Pharmacology
University of Pittsburgh
  School of Medicine
Pittsburgh, Pennsylvania*

Bruce R. Pitt, Ph.D.

*Vice Chairman, Department of Pharmacology
Professor of Pharmacology
  and Anesthesiology
University of Pittsburgh
  School of Medicine
Pittsburgh, Pennsylvania*

Joseph C. Glorioso, III, Ph.D.

*Chairman, Department of Molecular
  Genetics and Biochemistry
William S. McEllroy Professor of
  Biochemistry
University of Pittsburgh
  School of Medicine
Pittsburgh, Pennsylvania*

NMS

National Medical Series from Williams & Wilkins
Baltimore, Hong Kong, London, Sydney

Harwal Publishing Company, Malvern, Pennsylvania

The authors and publisher acknowledge with appreciation the use of questions from NMS books that exemplify the integrated format of the new examination.

The following illustrations have been reprinted with permission from the National Medical Series for Independent Study, Baltimore, Williams & Wilkins:
Figure 197–201, p 36, from April EW: *Anatomy,* 2nd edition, 1990
Figure 87, p 16, from Bullock J, Boyle J, Wang MB, et al: *Physiology,*1984
Figures 119, p 23, 127, p 24, 163, p 30, from Bullock J, Boyle J, Wang MB: *Physiology,* 2nd edition, 1991
Figures 13–15, p 3, 184–186, p 105, from Johnson KE: *Histology and Cell Biology,* 2nd edition, 1991
Figure 192–196, p 36, from Johnson KE: *Human Developmental Anatomy,* 1988

Figure 217–219, p 107, has been reprinted with permission from Sokolow M: *Clinical Cardiology,* 5th edition, East Norwalk, CT, Appleton & Lange, 1990
Figures 33, p 79, 153, p 27, and 141, p 97, have been reprinted with permission from Guyton AC: *Textbook of Medical Physiology,* 8th edition, Philadelphia, WB Saunders, 1991

Library of Congress Cataloging-in Publication Data

Lazo, John S.
    NMS review for NBME part I/USMLE step 1 examination /
John S. Lazo, Bruce R. Pitt, Joseph C. Glorioso, III. – 2nd ed.
        p.   cm. — (The National medical series for inde-
pendent study)
    Rev. ed. of: review for national board comprehensive part
I examination. c1991.
    ISBN 0-683-06209-3 (pbk.: alk. paper)
    1. Medicine—Examinations, questions, etc. I. Pitt, Bruce
R. II. Glorioso, Joseph C. III. Lazo, John S. Review for
national board comprehensive part I examination. IV. Title.
V Series.
    [DNLM: 1. Medicine—examination questions. W 18
L431ra]
R834.5.L38 1992
610'.76—dc20
DNLM/DLC
for Library of Congress   92-1469
                                            CIP

ISBN 0-683-06209-3

10 9 8 7 6 5 4 3 2

Dedication

To Jacqui, Shayna, and Stacy

Contents

Preface

Much like the events that took place during the first quarter of this century, there are major changes currently occurring in the approach to medical education in the United States. There have been rapid advances in our understanding of the molecular basis of diseases; an enormous increase in the data that can be presented to medical students; and a consolidation of experimental methodologies in the basic sciences. As a result, there is now a general consensus that a greater emphasis should be placed on an integrated presentation of information during the first 2 years of medical school.

Few institutions provide students with a comprehensive examination that will test their grasp of the key concepts presented in their first 2 years of medical school. With the advent of the new USMLE Step 1 that de-emphasizes the traditional basic science disciplines and stresses the integrated approach, we believe it is especially important to provide students with a series of questions that will prepare them for this new format. We hope you will find this book useful, and we, as well as the publisher, welcome any comments you may have.

John S. Lazo
Bruce R. Pitt
Joseph C. Glorioso, III

Acknowledgments

The writing of this book could not have been accomplished without the tremendous assistance of many individuals in the Departments of Pharmacology, Molecular Genetics and Biochemistry, and Human Genetics at the University of Pittsburgh. Particular thanks are extended to Drs. R. R. Bahnson, J. Barranger, A. Basu, C. Coffee, D. Edelstone, D. Feingold, W. F. Goins, E. P. Hoffman, D. Jaffurs, S. Kaplan, J. Lilja, M. Lotze, B. McClane, T. Mietzner, C. Milcarek, G. Morris, K. Norris, B. Phillips, S. Phillips, F. Ruben, S. Sebti, D. Tweardy, J. Yalowich, and S. Yousem. We also wish to acknowledge the contributions of John Mignano, Theresa Hartsell, and James Rusnak, who are medical students at the University of Pittsburgh, and Sharon Webb, for her secretarial support. Finally, this book could not have been successfully published without the thoughtful and tireless assistance of Jane Velker and Donna Siegfried at Harwal Publishing.

Publisher's Note

In 1983, the National Board of Medical Examiners created a study committee to review the format of the National Board exam and to evaluate its effectiveness vis-à-vis the current state of medical education. The committee identified a number of deficiencies in format and made some sweeping recommendations on how to improve the exam. In 1986, following the recommendations of the committee, the National Board appointed Comprehensive Part I and Comprehensive Part II committees and charged them with the responsibility of creating new examinations. The results became the National Board Comprehensive Part I and Part II exams. The Part I exam was introduced in June 1991. As of 1992, this test is called the United States Medical Licensing Examination (USMLE) Step 1.

The comprehensive exam differs from the old exam in both intent and format. The intent is best described by *The Medical Board Examiner* (Winter 1990).

(The new exam is) designed to be a broadly based, integrated examination for certification, rather than distinct achievement tests in individual basic science disciplines. Emphasis is on basic biomedical science concepts deemed important as part of the foundation for the current and future practice of medicine, including those related to the prevention of disease.

The format has been modified to reflect the objectives of the comprehensive exam. Concepts and information tested remain the same but are presented in a different framework. The new exam continues to use questions drawn from single disciplines but also includes questions designed to test whether the examinee understands and can apply concepts of basic biomedical science in an integrated, cross-discipline manner. Case studies, or vignettes, serve as clinical foundations for this approach.

The books in the National Medical Series (NMS) have always been exceptional sources of information for medical students. By using the narrative outline, the books facilitate learning a large amount of information in a short period of time. Whether they are used for course study, exam preparation, or Board review, the NMS books will continue to offer medical students a reliable low-cost way to excel.

This particular book on the NMS list is intended to be used along with the other NMS books and to help medical students:

- prepare for the USMLE Step 1 by reviewing all of the major content areas covered on the exam
- become acquainted and comfortable with the new exam format
- determine areas where they may need further study through the use of the key concepts included at the beginning of each explanation

Use this book along with other material as you prepare for the exam. The authors and publisher have made every effort to ensure that all of the information in this book is accurate. Best of luck.

The Publisher

Taking a Test

One of the least attractive aspects of pursuing an education is the necessity of being examined on what has been learned. Instructors do not like to prepare tests, and students do not like to take them.

However, students are required to take many examinations during their learning careers, and little if any time is spent acquainting them with the positive aspects of tests and with systematic and successful methods for approaching them. Students perceive tests as punitive and sometimes feel that they are merely opportunities for the instructor to discover what the student has forgotten or has never learned. Students need to view tests as opportunities to display their knowledge and to use them as tools for developing prescriptions for further study and learning.

A brief history and discussion of the National Board of Medical Examiners (NBME) examinations [now the United States Medical Licensing Examination (USMLE)] are presented here, along with ideas concerning psychological preparation for the examinations. Also presented are general considerations and test-taking tips, as well as ways to use practice exams as educational tools. (The literature provided by the various examination boards contains detailed information concerning the construction and scoring of specific exams.)

Before the various NBME exams were developed, each state attempted to license physicians through its own procedures. Differences in the quality and testing procedures of the various state examinations resulted in the refusal of some states to recognize the licensure of physicians licensed in other states. This made it difficult for physicians to move freely from one state to another and produced an uneven quality of medical care in the United States.

To remedy this situation, the various state medical boards decided they would be better served if an outside agency prepared standard exams to be given in all states, allowing each state to meet its own needs and have a common standard by which to judge the educational preparation of individuals applying for licensure.

One misconception concerning these outside agencies is that they are licensing authorities. This is not the case; they are examination boards only. The individual states retain the power to grant and revoke licenses. The examination boards are charged with designing and scoring valid and reliable tests. They are primarily concerned with providing the states with feedback on how examinees have performed and with making suggestions about the interpretation and usefulness of scores. The states use this information as partial fulfillment of qualifications upon which they grant licenses.

Students should remember that these exams are administered nationwide and, although the general medical information is the same, educational methodologies and faculty areas of expertise differ from institution to institution. It is unrealistic to expect that students will know all the material presented in the exams; they may face questions on the exams in areas that

The author of this introduction, Michael J. O'Donnell, holds the positions of Assistant Professor of Psychiatry and Director of Biomedical Communications at the University of New Mexico School of Medicine, Albuquerque, New Mexico.

were only superficially covered in their classes. The testing authorities recognize this situation, and their scoring procedures take it into account.

The Exams

The first exam was given in 1916. It was a combination of written, oral, and laboratory tests, and it was administered over a 5-day period. Admission to the exam required proof of completion of medical education and 1 year of internship.

In 1922, the examination was changed to a new format and was divided into three parts. Part I, a 3-day essay exam, was given in the basic sciences after 2 years of medical school. Part II, a 2-day exam, was administered shortly before or after graduation, and Part III was taken at the end of the first postgraduate year. To pass both Part I and Part II, a score equaling 75% of the total points available in each was required.

In 1954, after a 3-year extensive study, the NBME adopted the multiple-choice format. To pass, a statistically computed score of 75 was required, which allowed comparison of test results from year to year. In 1971, this method was changed to one that held the mean constant at a computed score of 500, with a predetermined deviation from the mean to ascertain a passing or failing score. The 1971 changes permitted more sophisticated analysis of test results and allowed schools to compare among individual students within their respective institutions as well as among students nationwide. Feedback to students regarding performance included the reporting of pass or failure along with scores in each of the areas tested.

During the 1980s, the ever-changing field of medicine made it necessary for the NBME to examine once again its evaluation strategies. It was found necessary to develop questions in multidisciplinary areas such as gerontology, health promotion, immunology, and cell and molecular biology. In addition, it was decided that questions should test higher cognitive levels and reasoning skills.

To meet the new goals, many changes have been made in both the form and content of the examination. Changes include reduction in the number of questions to approximately 800 in Step 1 and Step 2 of the USMLE to allow students more time on each question, with total testing time reduced on Step 1 from 13 to 12 hours and on Step 2 from 12.5 to 12 hours. The basic science disciplines are no longer allotted the same number of questions, which permits flexible weighing of the exam areas. Reporting of scores to schools includes total scores for individuals and group mean scores for separate discipline areas. Only pass/fail designations and total scores are reported to examinees. There is no longer a provision for the reporting of individual subscores to either the examinees or medical schools. Finally, the question format used in the new exams is predominately multiple-choice, best-answer.

The New Format

New questions, designed specifically for Step 1 are constructed in an effort to test the student's grasp of the sciences basic to medicine in an integrated fashion— the questions are designed to be interdisciplinary. Many of these items are presented as vignettes, or case studies, followed by a series of multiple-choice, best-answer questions.

The scoring of this exam is altered. Whereas in the past the exams were scored on a normal curve, the new exam has a predetermined standard, which must be met in order to pass. The exam no longer concentrates on the trivial; therefore, it has been concluded that there is a common base of information that all medical students should know in order to pass. It is anticipated that a major shift in the pass/fail rate for the nation is unlikely. In the past, the average student could only expect to feel comfortable with half the test and eventually would complete approximately 67% of the questions correctly, to achieve a mean score of 500. Although with the standard setting method it is likely that the mean score will change and become higher, it is unlikely that the pass/fail rates will differ significantly from those in the past. During the first testing in 1991, there was not differential weighing of questions. However, in the future, the NBME will be researching methods of weighing questions based on both the time it takes to answer questions vis-à-vis their difficulty and the perceived importance of the information. In addition, the NBME is attempting to design a method of delivering feedback to the student that will have considerable importance in discovering weaknesses and pinpointing areas for further study in the event that a retake is necessary.

Materials Needed for Test Preparation

In preparation for a test, many students collect far too much study material only to find that they simply do not have the time to go through all of it. They are defeated before they begin because either they leave areas unstudied, or they race through the material so quickly that they cannot benefit from the activity.

It is generally more efficient for the student to use materials already at hand; that is, class notes, one good outline to cover or strengthen areas not locally stressed and to quickly review the whole topic, and one good text as a reference for looking up complex material needing further explanation.

Also, many students attempt to memorize far too much information, rather than learning and understanding less material and then relying on that learned information to determine the answers to questions at the time of the examination. Relying too heavily on memorized material causes anxiety, and the more anxious students become during a test, the less learned knowledge they are likely to use.

Positive Attitude

A positive attitude and a realistic approach are essential to successful test taking. If concentration is placed on the negative aspects of tests or on the potential for failure, anxiety increases and performance decreases. A negative attitude generally develops if the student concentrates on "I must pass" rather than on "I can pass." "What if I fail?" becomes the major factor motivating the student to **run from failure rather than toward success.** This results from placing too much emphasis on scores rather than understanding that scores have only slight relevance to future professional performance.

The score received is only one aspect of test performance. Test performance also indicates the student's ability to use information during evaluation procedures and reveals how this ability might be used in the future. For example, when a patient enters the physician's office with a problem, the physician begins by asking questions, searching for clues, and seeking diagnostic information. Hypotheses are then developed, which will include several potential causes for the problem. Weighing the probabilities, the physician will begin to discard those hypotheses with the least likelihood of being correct. Good differential diagnosis involves the ability to deal with uncertainty, to reduce potential causes to the smallest number, and to use all learned information in arriving at a conclusion.

The same thought process can and should be used in testing situations. It might be termed **paper-and-pencil differential diagnosis.** In each question with five alternatives, of which one is correct, there are four alternatives that are incorrect. If deductive reasoning is used, as in solving a clinical problem, the choices can be viewed as having possibilities of being correct. The elimination of wrong choices increases the odds that a student will be able to recognize the correct choice. Even if the correct choice does not become evident, the probability of guessing correctly increases. Just as differential diagnosis in a clinical setting can result in a correct diagnosis, eliminating choices on a test can result in choosing the correct answer.

Answering questions based on what is incorrect is difficult for many students since they have had nearly 20 years experience taking tests with the implied assertion that knowledge can be displayed only by knowing what is correct. It must be remembered, however, that students can display knowledge by knowing something is wrong, just as they can display it by knowing something is right. **Students should begin to think in the present as they expect themselves to think in the future.**

Paper-and-Pencil Differential Diagnosis

The technique used to arrive at the answer to the following question is an example of the paper-and-pencil differential diagnosis approach.

A recently diagnosed case of hypothyroidism in a 45-year-old man may result in which of the following conditions?

(A) Thyrotoxicosis

(B) Cretinism

(C) Myxedema

(D) Graves' disease

(E) Hashimoto's thyroiditis

It is presumed that all of the choices presented in the question are plausible and partially correct. If the student begins by breaking the question into parts and trying to discover what the question is attempting to measure, it will be possible to answer the question correctly by using more than memorized charts concerning thyroid problems.

- The question may be testing if the student knows the difference between "hypo" and "hyper" conditions.
- The answer choices may include thyroid problems that are not "hypothyroid" problems.
- It is possible that one or more of the choices are "hypo" but are not "thyroid" problems, that they are some other endocrine problems.
- "Recently diagnosed in a 45-year-old man" indicates that the correct answer is not a congenital childhood problem.
- "May result in" as opposed to "resulting from" suggests that the choices might include a problem that **causes** hypothyroidism rather than **results from** hypothyroidism, as stated.

By applying this kind of reasoning, the student can see that choice **A**, thyroid toxicosis, which is a disorder resulting from an overactive thyroid gland ("hyper") must be eliminated. Another piece of knowledge, that is, Graves' disease is thyroid toxicosis, eliminates choice **D**. Choice **B**, cretinism, is indeed hypothyroidism, but is a childhood disorder. Therefore, **B** is eliminated. Choice **E** is an inflammation of the thyroid gland—here the clue is the suffix "itis." The reasoning is that thyroiditis, being an inflammation, may **cause** a thyroid problem, perhaps even a hypothyroid problem, but there is no reason for the reverse to be true. Myxedema, choice **C**, is the only choice left and the obvious correct answer.

Preparing for Board Examinations

1. Study for yourself. Although some of the material may seem irrelevant, the more you learn now, the less you will have to learn later. Also, do not let the fear of the test rob you of an important part of your education. If you study to learn, the task is less distasteful than studying solely to pass a test.

2. Review all areas. You should not be selective by studying perceived weak areas and ignoring perceived strong areas. This is probably the last time you will have the time and the motivation to review **all** of the basic sciences.

3. Attempt to understand, not just memorize, the material. Ask yourself: To whom does the material apply? Where does it apply? When does it apply? Understanding the connections among these points allows for longer retention and aids in those situations when guessing strategies may be needed.

4. Try to **anticipate questions that might appear on the test.** Ask yourself how you might construct a question on a specific topic.

5. Give yourself a couple days of rest before the test. Studying up to the last moment will increase your anxiety and cause potential confusion.

Taking Board Examinations

1. In the case of the USMLE, be sure to **pace yourself** to use the time optimally. Each booklet is designed to take 2 hours. You should use all of your allotted time; if you finish too early, you probably did so by moving too quickly through the test.

2. Read each question and all the alternatives carefully before you begin to make decisions. Remember the questions contain clues, as do the answer choices. As a physician, you would not make a clinical decision without a complete examination of all the data: the same holds true for answering test questions.

3. Read the directions for each question set carefully. You would be amazed at how many students make mistakes in tests simply because they have not paid close attention to the directions.

4. It is not advisable to leave blanks with the intention of coming back to answer the questions later. Because of the way Board examinations are constructed, you probably will not pick up any new information that will help you when you come back, and the chances of getting numerically off on your answer sheet are greater than your chances of benefiting by skipping around. If you feel that you must come back to a question, mark the best choice and place a note in the margin. Generally speaking, it is best not to change answers once you have made a decision. Your intuitive reaction and first response are correct more often than changes made out of frustration or anxiety. **Never turn in an answer sheet with blanks.** Scores are based on the number that you get correct; you are not penalized for incorrect choices.

5. Do not try to answer the questions on a stimulus-response basis. It generally will not work. Use all of your learned knowledge.

6. Do not let anxiety destroy your confidence. If you have prepared conscientiously, you know enough to pass. Use all that you have learned.

7. Do not try to determine how well you are doing as you proceed. You will not be able to make an objective assessment, and your anxiety will increase.

8. Do not expect a feeling of mastery or anything close to what you are accustomed to. Remember, this is a nationally administered exam, not a mastery test.

9. Do not become frustrated or angry about what appear to be bad or difficult questions. You simply do not know the answers; you cannot know everything.

Specific Test-Taking Strategies

Read the entire question carefully, regardless of format. Test questions have multiple parts. Concentrate on picking out the pertinent key words that might help you begin to problem-solve. Words such as "always," "never," "mostly," "primarily," and so forth play significant roles. In all types of questions, distractors with terms such as "always" or "never" most often are incorrect. Adjectives and adverbs can completely change the meaning of questions—pay close attention to them. Also, medical prefixes and suffixes (e.g., "hypo-," "hyper-," "-ectomy," "-itis") are sometimes at the root of the question. The knowledge and application of everyday English grammar often is the key to dissecting questions.

Multiple-Choice Questions

Read the question and the choices carefully to become familiar with the data as given. Remember, in multiple-choice questions there is one correct answer and there are four distractors, or incorrect answers. (Distractors are plausible and possibly correct or they would not be called distractors.) They are generally correct for part of the question but not for the entire question. Dissecting the question into parts aids in discerning these distractors.

If the correct answer is not immediately evident, begin eliminating the distractors. (Many students feel that they must always start at option A and make a decision before they move to B, thus forcing decisions they are not ready to make.) Your first decisions should be made on those choices you feel the most confident about.

Compare the choices to each part of the question. **To be wrong,** a choice needs to be **incorrect for only part** of the question. **To be correct,** it must be **totally** correct. If you believe a choice is partially incorrect, tentatively eliminate that choice. Make notes next to the choices regarding tentative decisions. One method is to place a minus sign next to the choices you are certain are incorrect and a plus sign next to those that potentially are correct. Finally, place a zero next to any choice you do not understand or need to come back to for further inspection. Do not feel that you must make final decisions until you have examined all choices carefully.

When you have eliminated as many choices as you can, decide which of those that are left has the highest probability of being correct. Remember to use paper-and-pencil differential diagnosis. Above all, be honest with yourself. If you do not know the answer, eliminate as many choices as possible and choose reasonably.

Vignette-Based Questions

Vignette-based questions are nothing more than normal multiple-choice questions that use the same case, or grouped information, for setting the problem. The NBME has been researching question types that would test the student's grasp of the integrated medical basic sciences in a more cognitively complex fashion than can be accomplished with traditional testing formats. These questions allow the testing of information that is more medically relevant than memorized terminology.

It is important to realize that several questions, although grouped together and referring to one situation or vignette, are independent questions; that is, they are able to stand alone. Your inability to answer one question in a group should have no bearing on your ability to answer other questions in that group.

These are multiple-choice questions, and just as with single best-answer questions, you should use the paper-and-pencil differential diagnosis, as was described earlier.

Single Best-Answer–Matching Sets

Single best-answer–matching sets consist of a list of words or statements followed by several numbered items or statements. Be sure to pay attention to whether the choices can be used more than once, only once, or not at all. Consider each choice individually and carefully. Begin with those with which you are the most familiar. It is important always to break the statements and words into parts, as with all other question formats. **If a choice is only partially correct, then it is incorrect.**

Guessing

Nothing takes the place of a firm knowledge base, but with little information to work with, even after playing paper-and-pencil differential diagnosis, you may find it necessary to guess at the correct answer. A few simple rules can help increase your guessing accuracy. Always guess consistently if you have no idea what is correct; that is, after eliminating all that you can, make the choice that agrees with your intuition or choose the option closest to the top of the list that has not been eliminated as a potential answer.

When guessing at questions that present with choices in numerical form, you will often find the choices listed in ascending or descending order. It is generally not wise to guess the first or last alternative, since these are usually extreme values and are most likely incorrect.

Using the USMLE to Learn

All too often, students do not take full advantage of practice exams. There is a tendency to complete the exam, score it, look up the correct answers to those questions missed, and then forget the entire thing.

In fact, great educational benefits can be derived if students would spend more time using practice tests as learning tools. As mentioned earlier, incorrect choices in test questions are plausible and partially correct or they would not fulfill their purpose as distractors. This means that it is just as beneficial to look up the incorrect choices as the correct choices to discover specifically why they are incorrect. In this way, it is possible to learn better test-taking skills as the subtlety of question construction is uncovered.

Additionally, it is advisable to go back and attempt to restructure each question to see if all the choices can be made correct by modifying the question. By doing this, four times as much will be learned. By all means, look up the right answer and explanation. Then, focus on each of the other choices and ask yourself under what conditions they might be correct. For example, the entire thrust of the sample question concerning hypothyroidism could be altered by changing the first few words to read:

> "Hyperthyroidism recently discovered in..."
> "Hypothyroidism prenatally occurring in..."
> "Hypothyroidism resulting from..."

This question can be used to learn and understand thyroid problems in general, not only to memorize answers to specific questions.

In the practice exams that follow, every effort has been made to simulate the types of questions and the degree of question difficulty in the USMLE Step 1. While taking these exams, the student should attempt to create the testing conditions that might be experienced during actual testing situations. Approximately 1 minute should be allowed for each question, and the entire test should be finished before it is scored.

Summary

Ideally, examinations are designed to determine how much information students have learned and how that information is used in the successful completion of the examination. Students will be successful if these suggestions are followed:

- Develop a positive attitude and maintain that attitude.
- Be realistic in determining the amount of material you attempt to master and in the score you hope to attain.
- Read the directions for each type of question and the questions themselves closely and follow the directions carefully.
- Guess intelligently and consistently when guessing strategies must be used.
- Bring the paper-and-pencil differential diagnosis approach to each question in the examination.
- Use the test as an opportunity to display your knowledge and as a tool for developing prescriptions for further study and learning.

The USMLE is not easy. It may be almost impossible for those who have unrealistic expectations or for those who allow misinformation concerning the exam to produce anxiety out of proportion to the task at hand. It is manageable if it is approached with a positive attitude and with consistent use of all the information that has been learned.

Michael J. O'Donnell

Practice Examination I

QUESTIONS

Directions: Each of the numbered items or incomplete statements in this section is followed by answers or by completions of the statement. Select the **one** lettered answer or completion that is **best** in each case.

1. In patients with Barrett's esophagus, factors responsible for the morphologic changes in the distal portion of the esophagus from normal squamous cell epithelium to columnar epithelium include all of the following EXCEPT

(A) incompetence of the lower esophageal sphincter
(B) the ingrowth of immature pluripotent stem cells
(C) increased exposure to acid and pepsin
(D) the absence of inflammatory processes
(E) increased exposure to bile acids and lysolecithin

2. Of the following effects, drug binding to plasma proteins generally

(A) limits glomerular filtration
(B) is highly drug-specific
(C) is an interaction between drug and immunoglobulins
(D) is irreversible
(E) limits renal tubular secretion

Questions 3–5

A 36-year-old woman is brought to the emergency room because she was found unresponsive on the floor of her home by a friend. Her friend relates a recent history of depression. An empty prescription bottle for 30 100-mg amitriptyline tablets was found nearby. The woman's amitriptyline level is 2300 ng/ml, and her serum ethanol level is 250 mg/100 ml.

3. The physician's first step would be to

(A) prepare involuntary commitment documents
(B) order an immediate electroencephalogram
(C) insert a nasogastric tube
(D) administer physostigmine
(E) place the patient on a respirator

The patient is placed on a cardiac monitor, the results of which are shown below.

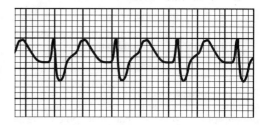

4. This electrocardiogram reveals which of the following patterns?

(A) Widened QRS complexes consistent with quinidine-like effects of tricyclics
(B) Bradycardia consistent with the cholinergic effects of tricyclics
(C) Premature ventricular contractions consistent with the toxic effects of ethanol
(D) S-T segment elevation consistent with the ischemic effects of ethanol
(E) Shortened P-R interval consistent with the toxic effects of tricyclics

5. The patient is now alert, her electrocardiogram is normal, and her total serum amitriptyline level is 128 ng/ml. The physician should next

(A) lecture her about the dangers of toxic doses of tricyclics
(B) elicit information about the suicide attempt
(C) interpret her behavior as an angry reaction
(D) discuss the paternalism of involuntary psychiatric hospitalization

6. The plasma membrane is composed of lipids and proteins with the basic structure of a lipid bilayer. Correct statements regarding the structure and function of the plasma membrane include all of the following EXCEPT

(A) phospholipids are amphipathic

(B) proteins may penetrate either portion of or the entire bilayer

(C) phospholipids promote free diffusion of ions and small water-soluble molecules

(D) proteins are amphipathic

(E) some large proteins are free to diffuse laterally in the plane of the membrane

7. A polymerase chain reaction can increase the sensitivity of certain genetic tests. Necessary components of a polymerase chain reaction include all of the following EXCEPT

(A) the DNA to be amplified is denatured in the presence of equimolar ratio of primers

(B) a heat-resistant DNA polymerase is used for strand synthesis

(C) multiple heating and cooling cycles are required for amplification of the DNA

(D) the sequence of the segment of DNA to which the primers will bind must be known

8. Of the following statements about messenger RNA (mRNA) transcription, the most accurate is that it

(A) proceeds by synthesis of the RNA in the 3' to 5' direction

(B) involves the removal of internal regions of DNA from the genome

(C) only occurs in the cytoplasm of the human cell

(D) may be regulated by hormones

(E) involves the post-transcriptional addition of adenylate nucleotides to the 5' end of the molecule

9. An individual with a gastric carcinoma is likely to present with any of the following skin lesions EXCEPT

(A) seborrheic keratosis

(B) acanthosis nigricans

(C) erythema nodosum

(D) amyloidosis

(E) Paget's disease

10. Which sequence below is the correct order of epidermal maturation?

(A) Stratum basale, stratum spinosum, stratum lucidum, stratum granulosum, stratum corneum

(B) Stratum basale, stratum spinosum, stratum granulosum, stratum lucidum, stratum corneum

(C) Stratum basale, stratum granulosum, stratum spinosum, stratum lucidum, stratum corneum

(D) Stratum basale, stratum lucidum, stratum spinosum, stratum granulosum, stratum corneum

(E) Stratum basale, stratum lucidum, stratum granulosum, stratum spinosum, stratum corneum

11. A 25-year-old sexually active woman is evaluated for her fourth acute urinary tract infection during the past 12 months. Her infections are characterized by frequency, urgency, dysuria, and *Escherichia coli* bacteriuria. Her recurrent infections are most likely due to

(A) overgrowth of highly resistant *E. coli* in her fecal reservoir

(B) passage of an infected renal calculus

(C) resistance of the bacteria to the drugs selected for treatment

(D) presence of a foreign body within the genitourinary tract

(E) colonization of the vaginal introitus with fecal Enterobacteriaceae

12. A 2-year-old child is hospitalized with splenomegaly, anemia, hypersplenism, hepatomegaly, and progressive nervous system dysfunction. Enzyme studies show an absence of glucocerebrosidase with an accumulation of β-glucosylceramide in macrophages and hepatocytes. The lipid storage disease most likely to be diagnosed in this child is

(A) Niemann-Pick disease

(B) Gaucher's disease, type II

(C) Krabbe's disease

(D) Tay-Sachs disease

Questions 13–15

The micrograph below is of the male reproductive system.

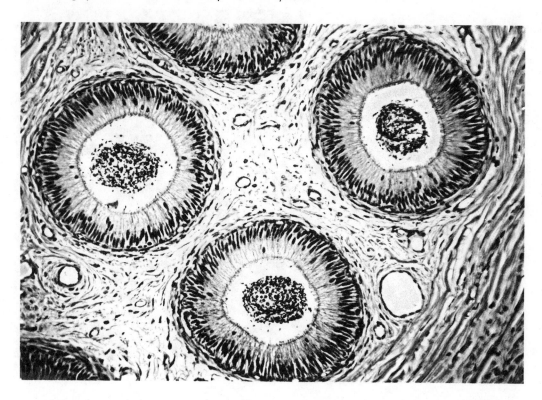

13. Which of the following organs is pictured in the micrograph?

(A) Testis
(B) Epididymis
(C) Vas deferens
(D) Seminal vesicle
(E) Bulbourethral gland

14. The epithelium of the organ pictured in the micrograph can best be described as

(A) simple cuboidal
(B) simple columnar
(C) stratified columnar
(D) pseudostratified columnar with stereocilia
(E) stratified squamous

15. Which adjective below best describes the function of the epithelium in the micrograph?

(A) Gametogenic
(B) Proliferative
(C) Secretory and absorptive
(D) Inactive
(E) Apoptotic

16. What condition is marked by formation of a malignant pustule?

(A) Enteritis necroticans
(B) Lockjaw
(C) Cutaneous anthrax
(D) Pseudomembranous colitis
(E) Woolsorter's disease

17. A 52-year-old man presented with painless swelling of his right testis. An orchiectomy was performed. A sample of the tissue is pictured in the photomicrograph below. The correct diagnosis is

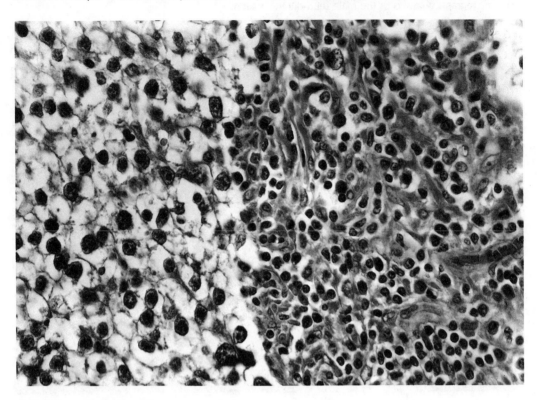

(A) seminoma

(B) mumps orchitis

(C) immature teratoma

(D) choriocarcinoma

18. A patient must be evaluated because of thrombocytopenia. The patient is a 55-year-old, previously well man, who was admitted to the hospital yesterday because of pneumonia. Antibiotic therapy was started, and his temperature continues to spike but is lower than on admission. On admission, his hemoglobin was reported to be 13 g/dl, white blood cell count was 9000/μl, and platelets 70,000/μl. The next laboratory study that should be done is

(A) bone marrow examination

(B) bleeding time

(C) examination of the peripheral smear

(D) platelet aggregation studies

(E) antiplatelet antibody detection tests

Questions 19–21

An infant is brought to the emergency room with severe oral thrush and hypocalcemia. A complete blood count shows a white cell count within normal limits. The mother admits to being an intravenous drug user.

19. What is the most likely diagnosis in this case?

(A) Chronic mucocutaneous candidiasis

(B) Severe combined immunodeficiency disease

(C) DiGeorge syndrome

(D) Chronic granulomatous disease

20. Which of the following statements concerning this child's condition is true?

(A) It is an autosomal recessive disorder
(B) It is an X-linked disorder
(C) It is the result of intrauterine damage
(D) The mode of inheritance is unknown

21. The most appropriate treatment for this patient would be

(A) transplantation of a fetal thymus
(B) infusion with white cells genetically engineered to produce adenosine deaminase
(C) administration of antifungal agents
(D) administration of corticosteroids

22. After osmotic equilibrium, infusion of several liters of a hypertonic saline solution will

(A) decrease intracellular osmolality
(B) not affect intracellular volume
(C) increase extracellular fluid volume
(D) decrease the plasma osmolarity

23. The Food and Drug Administration (FDA) has announced that it will test the vaccines against human immunodeficiency virus (HIV) with the least potential for causing the disease and the best chance of inducing protective immunity. Which of the vaccination reagents listed is most likely to be tested?

(A) An attenuated virus that does not cause disease in monkeys
(B) A recombinant HIV DNA in a vaccinia virus to induce host cells to produce only the HIV p24 protein, and then antibodies to p24 protein
(C) A denatured, purified CD4 (T4) protein to cause the host to mount an immune response to the HIV-infected $CD4^+$ cells
(D) A human monoclonal antibody that reacts with the intact CD4 (T4) receptor

24. All of the following statements concerning immunogenicity are true EXCEPT

(A) compounds with a molecular weight greater than 6000 daltons are generally immunogenic
(B) haptens become immunogenic only when coupled to high molecular weight carriers
(C) a homopolymer of lysine of molecular weight 30,000 daltons would not be immunogenic
(D) a polymer of lysine, methionine, and glutamate with a molecular weight of 10,000 daltons would not be immunogenic

25. The most important allosteric activator of glycolysis in the liver is which one of the following compounds?

(A) Fructose 2,6-bisphosphate
(B) Acetyl coenzyme A (acetyl CoA)
(C) Adenosine triphosphate (ATP)
(D) Citrate
(E) Glucose 6-phosphate

26. Ingestion of 150 mEq Na^+/day is usually balanced by excretion of a similar amount in urine. Since the glomerular filtrate normally contains 26,000 mEq Na^+/day, several important Na^+ reabsorbing mechanisms have evolved, including all of the following EXCEPT

(A) active transport of Na^+ from inside proximal epithelial cells to interstitial spaces
(B) passive cotransport of Na^+ with glucose or amino acids in the proximal tubular epithelium
(C) active transport in the thick segment of the loop of Henle
(D) hormone-independent passive reabsorption in the distal tubular epithelium

27. The thyroid tumor pictured here was removed from a 60-year-old woman whose medical history likely includes

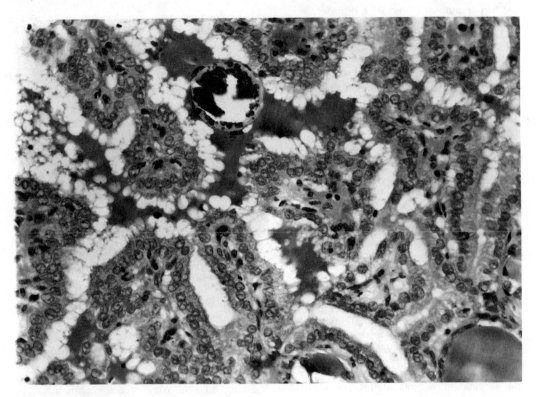

(A) hyperthyroidism
(B) hypothyroidism
(C) irradiation to the head and neck
(D) a pituitary adenoma

28. When comparing pertussis and diphtheria, true statements include which one of the following?

(A) Both pertussis and diphtheria are caused by bacteria that must adhere to respiratory tract cells
(B) Diphtheria symptoms are caused by an exotoxin, but no symptoms of pertussis result from an exotoxin
(C) The bacteria responsible for diphtheria and pertussis both produce endotoxin
(D) Pertussis is caused by an intracellular pathogen, but diphtheria is caused by an extracellular pathogen
(E) The neurologic problems observed with the current DTP (diphtheria-tetanus-pertussis) vaccine are caused by the diphtheria component of this vaccine

Questions 29–31

A 68-year-old widower complains of headaches, forgetfulness, decreased appetite, weight loss, insomnia, constipation, and anhedonia. An electrocardiogram shows first-degree heart block; he also has prostatic hypertrophy.

29. Considering side effect profiles, the best choice of medication would be

(A) imipramine
(B) phenelzine
(C) lithium carbonate
(D) clonazepam
(E) chlorpromazine

The patient's psychiatric symptoms improve with treatment, but his headaches persist. They occur daily and are bifrontotemporal, nonthrobbing, and bring him to tears when the pain is severe, but they do not disrupt his sleep. Physical examination reveals tenderness near the eye ridges.

30. The most appropriate test would be

(A) computed tomography scan of the head
(B) biopsy of the temporal artery
(C) electroencephalogram
(D) examination of the cerebrospinal fluid

31. Medication for migraine headache includes all of the following agents EXCEPT

(A) lithium carbonate
(B) ergotamine
(C) methysergide
(D) amitriptyline
(E) propranolol

32. Which of the following statements concerning the maturation of T cells is true?

(A) It occurs earliest in the thymic medulla
(B) It is independent of thymic epithelial cells
(C) It is independent of antigen
(D) None of the above

33. Each condition below is a diagnostically significant abnormality in Zellweger syndrome EXCEPT

(A) absent or grossly reduced numbers of peroxisomes
(B) catalase in the cytosol of hepatocytes
(C) overproduction of platelet activating factor (PAF)
(D) elevated plasma C26:0/C22:0 ratio
(E) accumulation of phytanic acid in central nervous system (CNS) tissues

34. A 24-year-old man presented to his family practitioner with a purulent penile discharge. Gonorrhea was diagnosed based upon the finding of intracellular gram-negative cocci in his discharge. He was given amoxicillin and probenecid. The infection improved, but 1 week later the patient still complained of a persistent urethral discharge and pain on urination. Upon a visit to a local clinic for sexually transmitted diseases, a diagnosis of postgonococcal urethritis was made. What is the most likely cause of his latest syndrome?

(A) A common side effect of probenecid administered during the initial treatment
(B) A lingering gonococcal infection caused by a penicillin-resistant strain of *Neisseria gonorrhoeae*
(C) An improper therapy regimen, which did not treat a coinciding chlamydial infection
(D) A side effect of the correct therapy regimen, which suppressed the patient's normal flora and allowed the establishment of a secondary infection

35. A 38-year-old man with AIDS develops meningitis. Microscopic examination of his spinal fluid shows yeast cells. India ink staining of these yeasts shows a visible clear halo surrounding each cell. Which one of the following pathogens is responsible for the man's meningitis?

(A) A virus
(B) *Cryptococcus neoformans*
(C) *Hemophilus influenzae*
(D) *Neisseria meningitidis*
(E) *Candida albicans*

36. All of the following properties are shared by acetylsalicylic acid (aspirin) and acetaminophen EXCEPT

(A) inhibits lipoxygenase activity
(B) analgesic activity
(C) antipyretic effects
(D) anti-inflammatory activity

37. Captopril is useful in the treatment of systemic hypertension because it

(A) blocks the effect of angiotensin II at its receptor in the central nervous system (CNS)

(B) directly relaxes vascular smooth muscle

(C) inhibits the movement of extracellular calcium into myocardial cells

(D) decreases the activity of angiotensin-converting enzyme (ACE)

(E) inhibits the production of renin

38. All of the following statements concerning insulin-dependent diabetes mellitus (type I; IDDM) are correct EXCEPT

(A) sulfonylureas may be a useful adjuvant to insulin therapy

(B) use of recombinant "human" insulin has eliminated problems of immunologic toxic effects

(C) insulin levels are routinely monitored

(D) ingestion of carbohydrates may be required to offset undesired hypoglycemia

(E) insulin therapy usually reverses the course of the disease

39. All of the following statements about allosteric enzymes are true EXCEPT

(A) positive cooperativity sensitizes the enzyme to small changes in substrate concentration

(B) they frequently catalyze the slowest step in a metabolic pathway

(C) the allosteric site can be located on a different subunit than the catalytic site

(D) the binding of a ligand to the allosteric site induces a conformational change in the active site

(E) they have substrate saturation curves that frequently show first-order kinetics

40. A patient presents with a torn medial collateral ligament of the left knee. Which of the following signs may be elicited on physical examination?

(A) Posterior displacement of the tibia

(B) Abnormal lateral rotation during extension

(C) Abnormal passive abduction of the extended leg

(D) Inability to lock the knee on full extension

41. The female reproductive viscera are best characterized by which of the following statements?

(A) The mesosalpinx contains the tubal branches of the uterine vessels

(B) The ovarian veins drain directly into the inferior vena cava

(C) Lymph from the cervix drains into the inguinal nodes

(D) Visceral afferent nerves from the body of the uterus course along the pelvic splanchnic nerves

42. The uterine cervical tissue shown in the photomicrograph below shows features of which one of the following infections?

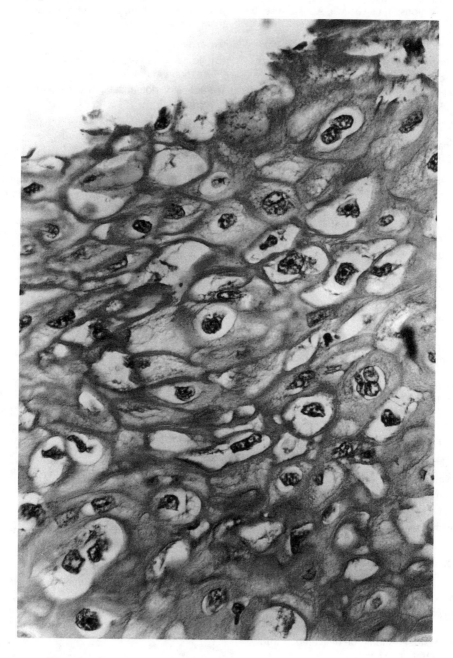

(A) Papilloma virus
(B) Herpes genitalis
(C) Gonorrheal cervicitis
(D) Carcinoma in situ

43. Tetracycline, a broad-spectrum antibiotic used in treating rickettsial, mycoplasmal, and chlamydial infections, receives widespread use because it

(A) is particularly useful in children
(B) causes minimal gastrointestinal side effects
(C) is bactericidal
(D) is selectively toxic to prokaryotes
(E) inhibits DNA-dependent RNA polymerase

44. Hepatic gluconeogenesis from alanine requires the participation of

(A) glucose 6-phosphatase and pyruvate kinase
(B) phosphofructokinase and pyruvate carboxylase
(C) pyruvate carboxylase and phosphoenolpyruvate carboxykinase
(D) fructose 1,6-diphosphatase and pyruvate kinase
(E) transaminase and phosphofructokinase

Questions 45–47

A resident has been assigned to the operating room for a 2-month rotation. The staff surgeon under whom he will work is a stickler for theory, and on the first day of the new rotation, he asked the resident the following questions.

45. With regard to anesthetics, MAC refers to

(A) maximum allowable concentration
(B) minimum alveolar concentration
(C) maximum alveolar concentration
(D) minimum arterial concentration
(E) maximum arterial concentration

46. If an anesthetic has a high blood:gas partition coefficient, it means that

(A) recovery will likely be prolonged
(B) lean patients should receive a lower dose than heavy patients
(C) the anesthetic should be delivered at a low concentration initially
(D) the anesthetic should be mixed with an inert gas or oxygen
(E) none of the above should occur

47. Nitrous oxide cannot be used alone to produce surgical anesthesia but is often used in conjunction with a more powerful agent, such as halothane, because nitrous oxide is

(A) explosive
(B) slow in onset of action due to a low blood:gas partition coefficient
(C) not very potent (i.e., has relatively low lipid solubility)
(D) rapidly metabolized

48. A 52-year-old middle school teacher has chronic peptic ulcer disease that has been treated for several years with ranitidine (Zantac) and metoclopramide (Reglan). On examination, the physician notes that the patient has involuntary, irregular chewing movements and repetitive tongue protrusion. The most likely cause of these movements is

(A) dystonic reaction
(B) Wilson's disease
(C) Huntington's disease
(D) cerebellar degeneration
(E) tardive dyskinesia

Questions 49–54

A mildly obese 20-year-old man presents to the emergency room at 5:00 A.M. He had ingested several six-packs of beer the evening before and had awakened at home with a sharp pain in his wrist at the radial–carpal articulation. The wrist is swollen and tender. The patient is slightly disoriented and ataxic but does not remember falling. X-rays of the wrist are negative. A slight fever is present.

49. The physician should order all of the following laboratory tests at this time EXCEPT

(A) synovial fluid analysis
(B) erythrocyte sedimentation rate
(C) C-reactive protein
(D) differential white blood cell count
(E) serum transaminase

50. Based on the data available, the most likely diagnosis is

(A) hyperuricemia with partial deficiency of hypoxanthine–guanine phosphoribosyltransferase
(B) Lesch-Nyhan syndrome
(C) osteoarthritis
(D) calcium hydroxyapatite deposition disease
(E) carpal tunnel syndrome

51. Synovial fluid analysis is done. The synovial fluid crystals are most likely composed of

(A) calcium oxalate
(B) calcium hydroxyapatite
(C) calcium carbonate
(D) sodium urate
(E) sodium oxalate

52. Biochemical studies confirm the suspected diagnosis. This patient suffers from lack of an enzyme whose product is

(A) 6-phosphogluconate
(B) citrulline
(C) inosinate
(D) oxaloacetate
(E) adenosine

53. The patient should be treated initially with

(A) adenosine replacement therapy
(B) azathioprine
(C) colchicine
(D) azidothymidine
(E) propoxyphene

54. For long-term therapy, the patient should be treated with

(A) acyclovir
(B) allopurinol
(C) amantadine
(D) acetazolamide
(E) ampicillin

55. Which of the following statements concerning primitive aortic arches and their derivatives is true?

(A) The left fourth aortic arch forms the arch of the aorta
(B) The right sixth aortic arch forms the right subclavian artery
(C) The left fifth aortic arch forms the ductus arteriosus
(D) The first aortic arch forms the common carotid artery

56. If forbidden clones are not deleted during T-cell development, a person may develop

(A) hypogammaglobulinemia
(B) a type I hypersensitivity reaction to exogenous antigens
(C) an autoimmune disease
(D) tolerance to autoantigens

57. A 60-year-old woman is brought to the hospital because of fever and confusion. One week ago, she received chemotherapy for lymphoma. In the emergency room, she is noted to have rapid breathing; cool, clammy skin; and a blood pressure of 70/40. Complete blood count shows a white blood cell count of $200/\mu l$. Gram stain of urine and sputum is negative. Which of the following empiric therapies would be most appropriate for this patient?

(A) Gentamicin
(B) Amikacin
(C) Chloramphenicol–gentamicin
(D) Piperacillin–gentamicin

Questions 58–60

A physician who has recommended urography for her competent, 68-year-old male patient is trying to decide whether or not to disclose the remote risk (1 in 10,000) of a fatal reaction.

58. If the physician favors nondisclosure, reasoning that it would not be in the patient's best interest to worry him with such remote risks, the physician is guided by

(A) beneficence but not nonmaleficence
(B) nonmaleficence but not beneficence
(C) both beneficence and nonmaleficence
(D) justice
(E) gratitude

59. If the physician believes that her decision should be determined by what other physicians would do in similar circumstances, she is guided by

(A) both beneficence and nonmaleficence
(B) strong paternalism
(C) weak paternalism
(D) respect for autonomy
(E) the professional practice standard

60. If the physician bases her decision on her assessment of whether or not the patient would want to learn about such remote risks, the physician is guided by

(A) respect for autonomy
(B) beneficence
(C) nonmaleficence
(D) both beneficence and nonmaleficence
(E) the professional practice standard

61. A scientist in the year 2350 is advising the NASA genetic engineering department concerning its attempts to engineer humans who can better survive the harsh climate of a planet that has high levels of ultraviolet (UV) light. The NASA engineers wish to incorporate a group of genes that will allow epidermal cells to produce a light-absorbing pigment. Of the following genetic manipulations, which would be most advantageous in cells in a UV-rich environment?

(A) Removal of intron DNA from the engineered genes

(B) Introducing the engineered genes in an overlapping fashion into the human genome

(C) Altering a theoretical human equivalent of the bacterial RecA protein in the cells to decrease its activity

(D) Producing genes with a low thymidine content

62. The photomicrograph below shows an adrenal mass, which was resected from a 2-year-old child. This lesion most likely is

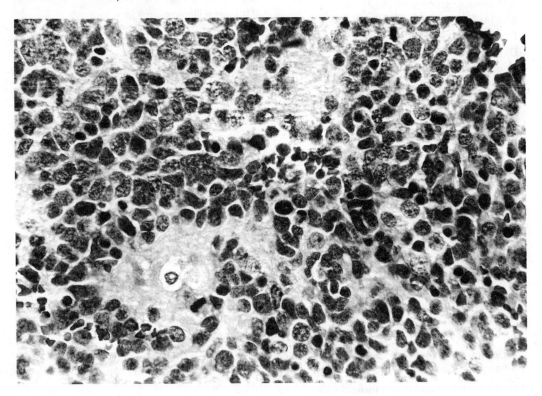

(A) Wilms' tumor

(B) a neuroblastoma

(C) a ganglioneuroma

(D) a pheochromocytoma

Questions 63–64

A 15-year-old girl presents for evaluation of short stature. She has not yet begun to menstruate. Examination reveals an intellectually normal child with short stature, webbing of neck, broad chest, and cubitus valgus.

63. Which of the following tests will provide the best evaluation of this patient?

(A) Amino acid analysis of urine

(B) Organic acid analysis of urine

(C) Serum long chain fatty acids

(D) Chromosome analysis

(E) Tissue glycogen content

64. The differential diagnosis for short stature would include all of the following disorders EXCEPT

(A) Klinefelter syndrome

(B) mucopolysaccharidoses

(C) gonadal dysgenesis

(D) progeria

65. Of the following amino acids, which one is released from skeletal muscle in amounts that exceed its relative abundance in muscle protein?

(A) Aspartate

(B) Alanine

(C) Glutamate

(D) Leucine

(E) Tyrosine

66. Rapid diagnosis and determination of the causal species is essential because of the immediately life-threatening nature of which one of the following parasitic infections?

(A) Malaria

(B) Chronic Chagas disease

(C) Amebic dysentery

(D) Mucocutaneous leishmaniasis

(E) Giardiasis

Questions 67–68

A patient weighing 50 kg is given a 20-mg/kg dose of a new drug. The plasma concentrations determined over time are illustrated in the graph below.

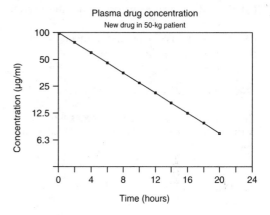

67. The drug's volume of distribution (V_d) is approximately

(A) 200 ml

(B) 1 L

(C) 2 L

(D) 10 L

(E) insufficient information to answer

68. The half-life of elimination of this drug is approximately

(A) 1 hour

(B) 2 hours

(C) 4 hours

(D) 10 hours

(E) insufficient information to answer

69. *N*-glycosylation of proteins occurs on which of the following amino acids?

(A) Asparagine

(B) Aspartate

(C) Lysine

(D) Serine

(E) Threonine

70. Tricyclic antidepressants (e.g., imipramine and amitriptyline) are useful agents for the management of endogenous depression because they

(A) reverse symptoms within days of initial administration
(B) have little effect on cardiovascular function
(C) affect dopamine receptors within the central nervous system (CNS)
(D) affect neuronal amine uptake mechanisms
(E) deplete brain serotonin levels

Questions 71–72

Cystic fibrosis is an autosomal recessive disease with an incidence of 1 per 1600 in the Caucasian population.

71. What is the frequency of the cystic fibrosis gene?

(A) 1/4
(B) 1/20
(C) 1/40
(D) 1/200
(E) 1/400

72. Of the following values, what proportion of the normal siblings of individuals with cystic fibrosis would most likely be carriers?

(A) 1/4
(B) 1/2
(C) 2/3
(D) All
(E) None

73. A 50-year-old woman with diabetes has an almost complete loss of renal function within 3 hours of a seemingly successful kidney transplant. All of the following statements concerning this type of rejection are true EXCEPT

(A) the patient had preformed antibodies to the graft
(B) the patient's rejection histologically resembles the classic Arthus reaction
(C) T cells are not directly involved
(D) administration of an immunosuppressive agent will restore kidney function

74. A 23-year-old woman with borderline personality disorder is hospitalized on a surgery ward to recover from fractures sustained in a motor vehicle accident. She complains that while her resident physician is wonderful and caring, her primary nurse is cold and cruel. The psychologic mechanism being displayed is best termed

(A) denial
(B) projection
(C) manipulation
(D) displacement
(E) splitting

75. Baroreceptors are highly branched nerve endings, which generate receptor potentials that are proportional to the rate of change in arterial blood pressure; they can also adapt to changes in arterial blood pressure over a prolonged period of time (hours to days). Which of the following statements concerning the specific properties of baroreceptors is most accurate?

(A) Baroreceptors are important for long-term regulation of blood pressure
(B) Clamping both carotid arteries after cutting both vagus nerves results in a decrease in arterial blood pressure
(C) Massaging the carotid sinus area leads to bradycardia and a decrease in arterial blood pressure
(D) A decrease in blood pressure activates baroreceptors, which, in turn, directly activate the vasomotor center

76. Lidocaine is the prototype of an amide local anesthetic and as such is

(A) free of potential central nervous system (CNS) side effects
(B) free of potential cardiac adverse effects
(C) rapidly metabolized by plasma cholinesterases
(D) a Na^+-channel blocker, especially in small, myelinated nerve fibers
(E) inappropriate for use in spinal anesthesia

77. Actin is a microfilament that is involved with all of the following activities EXCEPT

(A) endocytosis
(B) exocytosis
(C) cell locomotion
(D) mitotic spindle formation
(E) acrosome reaction

78. Mitochondria are important to the cells of eukaryotes for generating the adenosine triphosphate (ATP) necessary to carry out all energy-requiring processes. All of the following statements concerning mitochondria are true EXCEPT

(A) they contain a DNA molecule in a ring conformation

(B) mitochondrial proteins come solely from the cell nucleus

(C) the codons used by mitochondrial transfer RNA (tRNA) are not identical to those used in other mammalian genes

(D) mitochondrial proteins are encoded by gene sequences that overlap one another

79. A very painful, spreading, cutaneous edematous erythema is clinically descriptive of

(A) erysipeloid

(B) diphtheria

(C) Pontiac fever

(D) listeriosis

(E) nocardiosis

80. All of the following statements concerning gene duplication are true EXCEPT

(A) gene duplication involves unequal crossover between homologous repetitive DNA sequences during mitosis

(B) pseudogenes are nonfunctional duplications

(C) β-tubulins and β-like globins are perfect examples of duplicated gene families

(D) gene duplications are necessary to meet the cell's requirements for some RNA transcripts

81. Tay-Sachs disease occurs almost exclusively among Ashkenazi Jews, with an incidence of 1/3600. The frequency of carriers of the Tay-Sachs gene, which can be calculated by using the Hardy-Weinberg law ($p^2 + 2pq + q^2 = 1$), is which of the following?

(A) 1/4

(B) 1/30

(C) 1/60

(D) 1/600

(E) None of the above

82. Which of the endogenous substances listed is derived from the cyclooxygenase pathway of arachidonic acid metabolism?

(A) Platelet activating factor (PAF)

(B) Leukotriene D_4

(C) Eosinophil chemotactic factor (ECF)

(D) Thromboxane (TXA_2)

Questions 83–84

A 25-year-old medical student is buried by an avalanche of snow while skiing. Upon rescue, it is necessary to revive him from cardiopulmonary arrest. Although resuscitated, he remains in a coma for several hours before regaining consciousness.

83. It is known that the patient has suffered global hypoxia. The function most likely to have been lost under this condition is the ability to

(A) move facial muscles

(B) walk

(C) move arms

(D) move eyes

84. Which test of higher cortical functions would the patient most likely fail due to the hypoxic event?

(A) Remembering the name of the hospital or his physicians

(B) Reading a sentence

(C) Recognizing his cousins

(D) Adding two numbers together

85. A 65-year-old woman with degenerative joint disease secondary to rheumatoid arthritis has been admitted to the hospital for insertion of a prosthesis in her right hip (total hip arthroplasty). The physician is aware that *Staphylococcus aureus* and *Staphylococcus epidermidis* are likely to cause postoperative infection after total hip replacement. In addition, the hospital has reported a significant increase in beta-lactamase–resistant *S. aureus* isolates. Which of the following drugs is LEAST likely to be effective as prophylactic therapy in this patient?

(A) Cefazolin

(B) Methicillin

(C) Vancomycin

(D) Ampicillin

(E) Imipenem

86. A pregnant woman who is primigravida with blood type O-negative comes to the obstetrician's office for a routine visit. The patient states that her husband is AB-positive, and she is concerned about the incompatibility of the Rh factors. Her isohemagglutinin titers are normal. What would the most appropriate treatment be?

(A) Administer human anti-D globulin (RhoGAM) to the mother after the birth of the child

(B) Administer RhoGAM to the child immediately after birth

(C) Administer RhoGAM to the child if the blood is Rh-positive

(D) Do nothing at this time

87. In the figure below, the oxyhemoglobin dissociation curve is shown for a normal patient and for an anemic patient. A true statement concerning these patients is which one of the following?

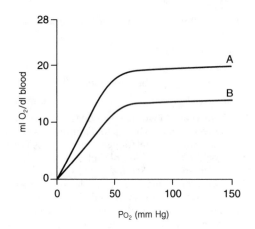

(A) Patient *A* is anemic

(B) Arterial Po_2 is likely to be similar for both subjects

(C) Venous Po_2 of the anemic subject will be greater than that of the normal subject at rest or during exercise

(D) If cardiac output is identical, then oxygen delivery will be identical in subjects *A* and *B*

88. A 45-year-old woman has eaten some home-canned vegetables. Two days later she has blurred vision and difficulty swallowing. This is followed by respiratory distress and flaccid paralysis. The symptoms of her illness result from an intoxication caused by a bacterial toxin whose action involves which one of the following effects?

(A) Adenosine diphosphate (ADP)-ribosylation of elongation factor 2

(B) Blockage of release of inhibitory neurotransmitters

(C) Blockage of release of acetylcholine (ACh)

(D) Stimulation of adenylate cyclase to elevate intracellular cyclic adenosine monophosphate (cAMP) levels

(E) Hemolysis resulting from sequestration of cholesterol in membranes

89. A 22-year-old woman reports the gradual onset and relentless progression of severe pain in the lower left quadrant of her abdomen. She also reported nausea with vomiting and fever. A pelvic exam determined that there was marked tenderness both upon direct palpation and upon manipulation of the cervix. A greenish-yellow discharge from the cervical os was noted, but a direct Gram stain of the discharge revealed no potential etiologic agents. Despite this finding, she was started on antibiotic therapy. Twenty-four hours later, laboratory culture of the discharge yielded growth of oxidase-positive, gram-negative diplococci on Thayer-Martin medium. A diagnosis of gonococcal salpingitis was made. One week post-therapy, the patient's symptoms were relieved and laboratory culture of her cervix revealed no pathogenic organisms. What is the patient's prognosis?

(A) The patient may not be cured and will require constant monitoring of her cervical flora for the next 6 months

(B) The patient may not be cured and is therefore encouraged to abstain from sexual encounters or observe safe-sex practices for the next 6 months

(C) The patient is cured and requires no further monitoring

(D) The patient is cured but faces an increased risk of subsequent episodes of pelvic inflammatory disease, infertility, and ectopic pregnancy

90. Which of the following structures contains Hassall's corpuscles?

(A) Thyroid gland
(B) Parathyroid gland
(C) Pineal gland
(D) Thymus
(E) Spleen

91. Synthesis of glycogen from fructose in a person with essential fructosuria requires the activity of which one of the following enzymes?

(A) Transketolase
(B) Aldolase B
(C) Hexokinase
(D) Fructokinase
(E) Glucokinase

92. Renal osteodystrophy is a condition that may follow chronic renal failure. Features of this condition include osteitis fibrosa cystica admixed with osteomalacia. The pathogenesis of this condition is characterized by all of the following EXCEPT

(A) phosphate retention and hyperphosphatemia
(B) low levels of 1,25-dihydroxyvitamin D_3 (calcitriol)
(C) elevated levels of calcitonin
(D) hyperparathyroidism
(E) hypocalcemia

93. A 65-year-old woman is seen prior to cataract surgery. She has had no previous surgery except for a dental extraction, after which she bled for 10 days and required a 2-unit blood transfusion. One sibling died from postoperative hemorrhage during childhood, and there is a history of bleeding in a number of relatives, both male and female. Her partial thromboplastin time (PTT) is markedly prolonged, and the bleeding time is within normal limits. The most likely diagnosis is

(A) factor VIII deficiency
(B) factor XI deficiency
(C) factor XII deficiency
(D) Fletcher factor deficiency
(E) von Willebrand's disease

94. Enteric pathogens vary with respect to their ability to invade the intestinal mucosa. After infection, which one of the following enteric pathogens is most likely to invade the intestinal submucosa and then disseminate throughout the body?

(A) *Vibrio cholerae*
(B) *Salmonella typhi*
(C) *Shigella dysenteriae*
(D) Nontyphoid *Salmonella*
(E) *Campylobacter jejuni*

Questions 95–96

A 45-year-old woman is admitted to the hospital with an unremitting sore throat. She has undergone radical mastectomy for breast carcinoma and recently underwent adjuvant chemotherapy. Two weeks before, she received a seven-day course of amoxicillin–clavulanic acid (Augmentin) for a recurrent urinary tract infection. Examination of her palate reveals several patches of white, creamy, curd-like friable lesions on the tongue and other mucosal surfaces.

95. This patient most likely has which type of fungal infection?

(A) Sporotrichosis
(B) Dermatomycosis
(C) Candidiasis
(D) Cryptococcosis

96. All the following therapies would be effective for this fungal infection EXCEPT

(A) ketoconazole
(B) oral fluconazole
(C) topical nystatin
(D) oral griseofulvin
(E) clotrimazole

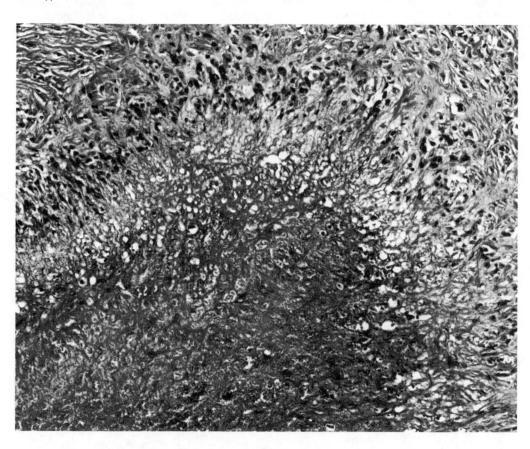

97. An elderly woman had a synovial biopsy and total knee replacement for degenerative joint disease. Sections of the synovium revealed the findings shown in the above photomicrograph, indicating a history of which one of the following conditions?

(A) Colchicine therapy for gout
(B) Repeated fractures
(C) Rheumatoid arthritis
(D) Trauma and foreign body the joint space

98. Pictured below is a portion of large bowel resected from a middle-aged woman who had repeated bouts of crampy abdominal pain. It would be concluded from the histology that the gross appearance of the bowel would show all of the following features EXCEPT

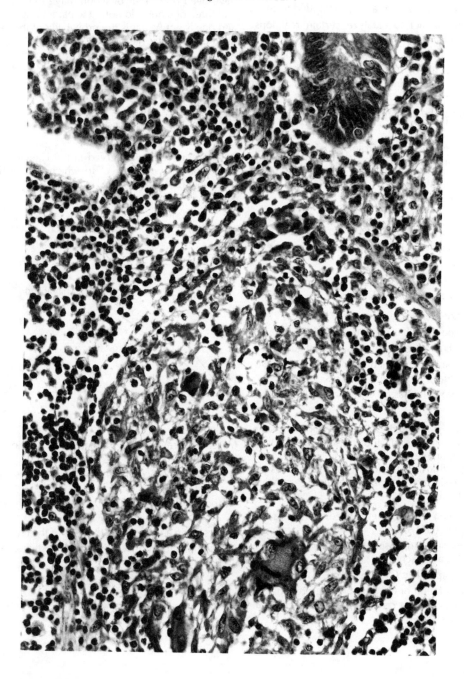

(A) segmental lesions
(B) "creeping fat"
(C) a thickened wall
(D) pseudopolyps
(E) long, snake-like lesions

99. All of the following statements about RNA are true EXCEPT

(A) RNA occurs only in a single-stranded form
(B) RNA can act to catalyze certain reactions, much like an enzyme
(C) RNA can act as primary genetic material
(D) a molecule of RNA differs from DNA in the number of hydroxyl groups present on the sugar moieties
(E) none of the above

100. Cimetidine is the prototype of a histamine receptor antagonist that

(A) causes sedation
(B) is useful for motion sickness
(C) enhances hepatic drug-metabolizing enzymes
(D) reduces gastric acid secretion
(E) is useful in the treatment of certain allergies

101. All of the following statements about the peptide bond are true EXCEPT the

(A) peptide bond is planar
(B) peptide bond has restricted rotation
(C) α-carbon atoms are in a *trans* configuration
(D) peptide bond atoms do not participate in the secondary structure of proteins
(E) peptide bond has no charge associated with it

102. Ca^{2+} is required for various processes, such as neurotransmission and muscle contraction. However, an elevated level of Ca^{2+} can be cytotoxic to cells. All of the following mechanisms are used by cells to regulate intracellular Ca^{2+} concentration EXCEPT

(A) chelation of Ca^{2+} by ethylenediaminetetraacetic acid (EDTA)
(B) adenosine triphosphate (ATP)-independent Na^+–Ca^{2+} exchange
(C) ATP-dependent Ca^{2+} pumping
(D) sequestration of Ca^{2+} by binding proteins
(E) sequestration of Ca^{2+} in the endoplasmic reticulum

103. In a family with a disease that has an autosomal dominant inheritance pattern, seven children have been born, four of whom have the disease and three of whom do not. One parent is affected and one is not. What is the probability of the next child born having the disease?

(A) 100%
(B) 50%
(C) 25%
(D) Zero
(E) Cannot be determined

104. The inhibition observed in the Lineweaver-Burk plot below is subject to which one of the following actions? It

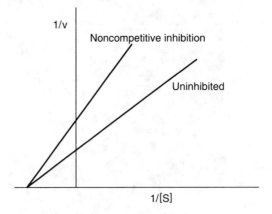

(A) can be reversed by a high concentration of substrate
(B) results from compounds that are transition-state analogs
(C) occurs through the interaction of the inhibitor at the active site
(D) results in a decrease in the V_{max} of the reaction
(E) is characterized by an increase in the K_m for the substrate

105. All of the following statements about the protein kinase C signal transduction pathway are true EXCEPT

(A) after activation, protein kinase C is degraded to protein kinase M
(B) protein kinase C phosphorylates tyrosines on proteins
(C) protein kinase C requires Ca^{2+} for full activation
(D) protein kinase C requires lipids for full activation
(E) protein kinase C is translocated to the plasma membrane

106. A patient is on a ventilator. The patient's anatomic dead space is 150 ml, and the ventilator's dead space is 250 ml. The ventilatory rate is set at 20 per minute. What should the output (tidal volume) of the ventilator be adjusted to so that alveolar minute ventilation is 4 L/min?

(A) 150 ml
(B) 250 ml
(C) 400 ml
(D) 600 ml
(E) 1000 ml

107. Each statement below concerning fenestrated capillaries is true EXCEPT

(A) fenestrations are 60 nm to 100 nm in diameter
(B) they are present in the choroid plexus
(C) they may be partially surrounded by pericytes
(D) they are present in endocrine glands
(E) they have a slit diaphragm that forms a filtration barrier in the renal glomerulus

108. Pathogenic bacteria enter the body by various routes, and entry mechanisms are critical for understanding the pathogenesis and transmissibility of each agent. Which one of the following is a correct association between a pathogen and its common entry mechanism?

(A) *Neisseria meningitidis* — sexually transmitted entry
(B) *Corynebacterium diphtheriae* — food-borne entry
(C) *Rickettsia rickettsii* — entry by contamination of wound with soil
(D) *Clostridium tetani* — inhalation entry
(E) *Borrelia burgdorferi* — arthropod vector–borne entry

Questions 109–111

A 70-year-old man is brought to the hospital, and a neurologist is called for a consultation. The residents caring for the patient tell the physician that he has spastic paralysis on one side of his body but has no sensory deficit.

109. On examination, the physician finds that the patient can move neither the right side of his face nor his left extremities. He has right-sided ptosis of the eyelid, and the right eye deviates laterally. The right eye also does not respond to light or exhibit accommodation. What is the most likely site of the patient's lesion?

(A) The midbrain
(B) The pons
(C) The medulla
(D) None of the above

110. The lesion is most likely a cerebral vascular accident, resulting in occlusion of which one of the following arteries?

(A) Basilar artery
(B) Middle cerebral artery
(C) Posterior cerebral artery
(D) Superior cerebellar artery

111. After examining the patient, the physician is most likely to propose which of the following syndromes in his evaluation?

(A) Millard-Gubler syndrome
(B) Weber's syndrome
(C) Brown-Séquard syndrome
(D) None of the above

112. Each statement below concerning cyclic adenosine monophosphate (cAMP) is true EXCEPT

(A) cAMP levels may be increased or decreased by hormone stimulation
(B) it is the second messenger for the action of parathyroid hormone (PTH) on the kidney
(C) it activates protein kinase C by binding to the regulatory subunit and causing dissociation of the catalytic subunit
(D) it is degraded intracellularly by a family of phosphodiesterase isoenzymes
(E) it is synthesized from adenosine triphosphate (ATP)

113. Which one of the following statements about glycogen storage disease type Ia is true?

(A) Liver glycogen is decreased
(B) Renal glycogen is increased
(C) Phosphorylase A is deficient
(D) Debranching enzyme is deficient
(E) None of the above

114. Tay-Sachs disease is marked by all of the following EXCEPT

(A) it is more common among Ashkenazi Jews than other population groups
(B) it is a lysosomal storage disease
(C) it is characterized by an absence of hexosaminidase A
(D) it is characterized by an accumulation of GM_2 gangliosides
(E) it is characterized by an absence of β-galactosidase

Questions 115–118

A patient complains of chest pains that are appreciable upon exercise. Electrocardiogram, stress scintigraphy, and coronary arteriography indicate that the patient has typical (exertional) angina pectoris due to atherosclerotic coronary artery disease.

115. Which of the following statements regarding coronary artery blood flow in a healthy person is true?

(A) During systole, coronary artery blood flow is uniform from subendocardial to epicardial regions of the left ventricle
(B) Myocardial oxygen extraction, not coronary artery blood flow, increases during exercise
(C) Coronary artery blood flow is directly proportional to arterial blood pressure over a range of pressures within 20–30 torrs of normal
(D) Coronary artery blood flow is proportional to myocardial oxygen demands
(E) Coronary artery blood flow is maximal during systole

116. Initial pharmacotherapy for the patient includes nitroglycerin, sublingually, at the onset of chest pain. Relaxation of vascular smooth muscle by nitroglycerin is due to its metabolism to an intermediate that is similar in structure and activity to

(A) nitrogen dioxide
(B) nitrous oxide
(C) nitric oxide
(D) cyanide
(E) thiocyanate

117. Continued use of nitroglycerin causes profound hypotension and an increase in heart rate, which is likely to be

(A) a reflex originating from aortic and carotid baroreceptors
(B) a direct effect of nitroglycerin in cardiac pacemaker cells
(C) an atriopeptin-mediated effect originating from myocytes of the left atrium
(D) a direct effect of nitroglycerin on the central nervous system (CNS)
(E) an indirect effect of nitroglycerin via its positive chronotropic effect on the heart

118. A useful adjuvant to minimize the nitroglycerin-associated tachycardia is

(A) enalapril
(B) hexamethonium
(C) atropine
(D) isoproterenol
(E) propranolol

119. An action potential recorded from a microelectrode inserted in a nerve fiber is illustrated in the figure below. All of the following statements describe changes that take place during the action potential recorded by this electrode EXCEPT

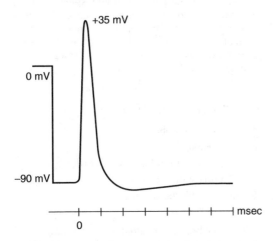

(A) at the peak of the action potential, the number of open Na$^+$ channels greatly exceeds the number of open K$^+$ channels

(B) depolarization is due to an abrupt increase in Na$^+$ conductance

(C) repolarization is primarily due to an increase in K$^+$ conductance

(D) repolarization is due to activation of the Ca^{2+}–Na$^+$ channel

(E) chloride channel permeability does not change during an action potential

120. A 35-year-old black male presents with loss of pain sensation in the skin of the forearm and lateral border of the leg. He also exhibits loss of tendon reflexes and complains of severe stabbing pains of the legs. This condition could have been prevented by

(A) avoiding the bullet that damaged his cingulate gyrus 13 years ago

(B) early penicillin treatment

(C) avoiding exposure to varicella zoster virus infection

(D) early administration of acyclovir

121. All of the following statements concerning the major determinants of glomerular filtration rate (GFR), which are renal blood flow (RBF) and glomerular hydrostatic pressures, are correct EXCEPT

(A) constriction of the afferent arteriole decreases both RBF and GFR

(B) an increase in RBF, even with little change in glomerular pressure, increases GFR

(C) in a normal kidney, an increase in systemic arterial pressure from 100 to 150 mm Hg increases GFR severalfold

(D) constriction of the efferent arteriole decreases RBF and slightly increases GFR

122. At which of these blood neutrophil levels do patients acquire a significant risk of opportunistic infection?

(A) < 1000/μl
(B) 1000 – 1500/μl
(C) 1500 – 2000/μl
(D) 2000 – 2500/μl
(E) 2500 – 3000/μl

123. A physician interested in evaluating the effects of a drug on the synthesis of RNA has decided to measure RNA production in cells after treatment with the drug by radiolabeling RNA. Which of the following radiolabeled bases should this physician use?

(A) Tritiated thymine [(^{3}H)-thymine]
(B) Tritiated guanine [(^{3}H)-guanine]
(C) Tritiated adenine [(^{3}H)-adenine]
(D) Tritiated uracil [(^{3}H)-uracil]
(E) Tritiated cytosine [(^{3}H)-cytosine]

124. Of the following statements, which best describes integral membrane proteins? They

(A) have at least one α-helical domain of approximately 20 amino acids, which spans the bilayer

(B) are stabilized within the bilayer by a combination of hydrogen bonds and electrostatic interactions

(C) may be solubilized by altering the pH or the ionic strength

(D) are frequently glycoproteins in which the carbohydrate is on the cytosolic side of the membrane

(E) may display transverse movement in the lipid bilayer

125. For a patient trying to prevent intercourse-related recurrent urinary tract infections, which of the following antibiotics would be the most effective and economical when administered only once after coitus?

(A) Cephalexin

(B) Nitrofurantoin

(C) Trimethoprim–sulfamethoxazole

(D) Ciprofloxacin

(E) Penicillin G

126. For which one of the following organisms do opsonic antibodies play a major role in acquired immunity to infection?

(A) *Neisseria meningitidis,* group A

(B) *Vibrio cholerae*

(C) *Clostridium botulinum*

(D) *Shigella flexneri*

127. If end diastolic volume is approximately 115 ml in the volume–pressure curve of the left ventricle below, then which of the following statements is most accurate?

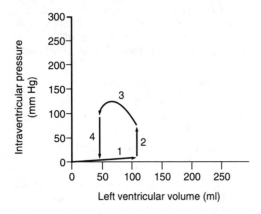

(A) The ejection fraction is approximately 30%

(B) Aortic diastolic pressure is approximately 80 mm Hg

(C) Isovolumic contraction is during the section labeled *3*

(D) Stroke volume is approximately 45 ml

(E) Left ventricular end diastolic pressure is approximately 100 mm Hg

Questions 128–130

A 45-year-old man has complained of increasing abdominal girth, fever, and malaise for the previous 4 months; he has denied cough. Physical examination shows a markedly enlarged spleen but no lymphadenopathy. Laboratory evaluation reveals a normal chest x-ray, hemoglobin concentration of 15 g/dl, a white blood cell count of 45,000 cells/μl with no blasts seen on the blood smear, and a platelet count of 750,000/μl.

128. The most likely diagnosis is

(A) malignant lymphoma

(B) acute leukemia

(C) chronic myeloproliferative disorder

(D) pulmonary tuberculosis

(E) myelodysplastic disorder

129. The laboratory evaluation for the differential diagnosis of this problem might include all of the following tests EXCEPT

(A) measurement of leukocyte alkaline phosphatase levels

(B) chromosomal evaluation

(C) bone marrow aspiration and biopsy

(D) flow cytometric analysis

(E) determination of red blood cell mass

130. Evaluation of chromosomes reveals a normal male karyotype. The leukocyte alkaline phosphatase level is low–normal, and the bone marrow is hypercellular and shows a myeloid-to-erythroid cell ratio of 10:1. Of the following conclusions, which is most appropriate?

(A) Chronic myelogenous leukemia (CML) is excluded, and the patient has a leukemoid reaction

(B) CML is excluded; therefore, the patient has an excellent prognosis and will be monitored every 6 months

(C) CML is excluded, and further workup will differentiate polycythemia vera from agnogenic myeloid metaplasia

(D) CML has not been excluded and further workup should include a molecular examination for a BCR-*abl* proto-oncogene translocation

131. Chronic Chagas disease should be considered in patients from Central and South America presenting with which set of the following signs and symptoms?

(A) Periodic fever and chills

(B) Cardiac conduction defects

(C) Multiple mucocutaneous lesions

(D) Persistent diarrhea

(E) Pneumonia

Questions 132–139

A 27-year-old woman presents with muscle weakness, including eyelid ptosis, slurred speech, and difficulty swallowing. The history reveals that the woman is being treated for a gram-negative infection with gentamicin. The following tests have been ordered: thyroid function studies, serum creatine kinase, an electromyogram, and a muscle biopsy.

132. The attending physician chides the resident on the case for not ordering edrophonium, which produces a dramatic improvement in the patient's muscle strength when administered intravenously. All of the other tests that were ordered returned with normal values. The resident's working diagnosis is

(A) Duchenne muscular dystrophy (DMD)

(B) monoadenylate deaminase deficiency

(C) myasthenia gravis

(D) hyperthyroidism

(E) toxic drug myopathy

133. This patient's condition most likely results from

(A) inadequate acetylcholinesterase in the synaptic cleft

(B) production of defective acetylcholine (ACh) receptors

(C) impaired synthesis or storage of ACh in presynaptic vesicles

(D) impaired release of ACh from presynaptic terminals

(E) blockade and increased turnover of ACh receptors

134. Aminoglycoside antibiotics create and exacerbate muscle weakness through

(A) inhibition of presynaptic release of ACh

(B) antagonism of the action of acetylcholinesterase

(C) potentiation of the action of acetylcholinesterase

(D) increasing the turnover of ACh receptors

(E) slowing conduction of the action potential

135. The adverse effects of the aminoglycoside antibiotics can be overcome with the intravenous administration of

(A) magnesium gluconate

(B) calcium gluconate

(C) magnesium phosphate

(D) copper sulfate

(E) creatine phosphate

136. Besides the aminoglycosides, another drug known to create muscle weakness is

(A) imipenem

(B) actinomycin

(C) tetracycline

(D) penicillamine

(E) amoxicillin

137. A more thorough physical examination of this patient would likely reveal an abnormal

(A) adrenal

(B) heart

(C) kidney

(D) thymus

(E) thyroid

138. Primary treatment of this patient's condition should begin with

(A) isoflurophate (di*iso*propyl phosphorofluoridate; DFP)

(B) mefenamic acid

(C) pralidoxime

(D) pyridostigmine

(E) triorthocresylphosphate

139. Long-term treatment should also include

(A) echothiophate

(B) edrophonium

(C) glucocorticoids

(D) succinylcholine

(E) vitamin and mineral supplementation

140. A hospitalized patient is noted to have a urinary tract infection due to *Serratia*. A course of antimicrobial therapy with an aminoglycoside is planned. However, the patient is noted to have mild renal impairment. The best means to determine the appropriate drug dosage is

(A) body surface area

(B) serum creatinine

(C) serum blood urea nitrogen

(D) creatinine clearance

(E) peak and trough drug levels

141. All of the following match important vasodilators with corresponding tissues EXCEPT

(A) adenosine–heart

(B) carbon dioxide–brain

(C) low oxygen–lung

(D) increased body temperature–skin

142. Surgical instruments are boiled for 10 minutes in a saline solution containing *Escherichia coli, Mycobacterium tuberculosis,* and *Bacillus cereus*. Which one of the following organisms is most likely to survive this procedure?

(A) *E. coli*

(B) *M. tuberculosis*

(C) *B. cereus*

Questions 143–144

A 68-year-old woman suddenly develops a fever of 38.2° C and a severe headache one evening. The following morning she also experiences a stiff neck and uncharacteristic drowsiness. At the emergency room, her temperature is 38.8° C, and there is pain and resistance on flexion of her neck. The patient is noted to be mentally competent although lethargic. A cerebral spinal fluid sample is obtained by lumbar puncture.

143. On the basis of the history and physical examination of this patient, what is the most probable diagnosis?

(A) Viral meningitis

(B) Fungal meningitis

(C) Bacterial meningitis

(D) Viral encephalitis

(E) Brain abscess

144. On the basis of the patient's age, the probable etiologic agent is

(A) *Staphylococcus aureus*

(B) *Hemophilus influenzae*

(C) *Streptococcus pneumoniae*

(D) *Neisseria meningitidis*

(E) none of the above

Questions 145–146

A 35-year-old man contracts something resembling the flu, receives no treatment, and is sick for a few days. Three and one-half weeks later, he develops "a feeling of pins and needles" in his fingers and toes. Three days after that he has trouble speaking and eating, and he keeps cutting the right side of his face while shaving because "it is numb." The next day, upon waking, he has trouble with his gait. He goes to the hospital, and he tells the physician that he has never been ill before in his life. He is barely able to lift his arms to a horizontal position, and he cannot walk well. All of his tendon reflexes are absent.

145. Which one of the following diseases is the patient most likely to have?

(A) Myasthenia gravis

(B) Polio

(C) Guillain-Barré syndrome

(D) Raynaud's phenomenon

146. This disease is thought to be caused by

(A) destruction of anterior horn cells due to picornavirus infection

(B) autoantibodies to the acetylcholine (ACh) receptors

(C) damage to spinal nerves

(D) peripheral arteriosclerosis

147. Agnogenic myeloid metaplasia with myelofibrosis is characterized by all of the following features EXCEPT

(A) hypocellular bone marrow

(B) normal levels of leukocyte alkaline phosphatase

(C) teardrop-shaped erythrocytes

(D) hepatomegaly

(E) splenomegaly

148. All of the following characteristics of warfarin are accurate EXCEPT

(A) it is useful in pregnant women because it does not cross the placenta
(B) it affects hepatic synthesis of clotting factors present in blood
(C) it is effective after oral administration
(D) it is primarily used in chronic therapy
(E) therapy can be reversed by administration of vitamin K

149. A patient hospitalized for multiple fractures was placed on a prophylactic antibiotic. Two days prior to discharge, diarrhea developed, requiring intravenous rehydration. The antibiotic was changed to a broad-spectrum cephalosporin, but diarrhea continued and the patient's condition deteriorated. All of the following actions are appropriate EXCEPT

(A) sigmoidoscopic examination
(B) proper isolation of the patient
(C) Gram stain of feces for white blood cells
(D) a request for *Clostridium difficile* toxin test
(E) changing the antibiotic to clindamycin

150. Low levels of cellular 3-hydroxy-3-methyl-glutaryl coenzyme A (HMG CoA) reductase activity in humans is most likely to result from

(A) a vegetarian diet
(B) the administration of a bile acid–sequestering resin
(C) familial hypercholesterolemia
(D) a long-term high cholesterol diet

151. Which one of the following fatty acids found in a normal diet is metabolized by the α-hydroxylase pathway?

(A) Linoleic acid
(B) Phytanic acid
(C) Arachidonic acid
(D) Palmitic acid
(E) Decenoic acid

152. All of the following statements describe the biologic properties of immunoglobulin E (IgE) EXCEPT

(A) it has the shortest half-life of all classes of immunoglobulins
(B) low levels of circulating IgE are due in part to the high-affinity binding of the Fc portion to mast cells and basophils
(C) it can cause agglutination of particulate antigens
(D) it is elevated in cases of certain parasitic infections

153. A length–tension diagram for a single sarcomere is illustrated below. Tension that develops is maximal between points *B* and *C* because

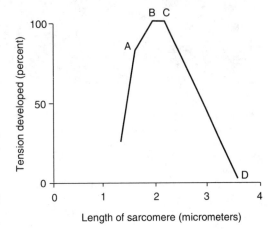

Length of sarcomere (micrometers)

(A) there is maximal overlap between the actin filaments and the cross-bridges of the myosin filaments
(B) the actin filament has pulled all the way out to the end of the myosin filament
(C) the Z disks of the sarcomere touch the ends of the myosin filament
(D) the myosin filament is at its minimal length
(E) actin filaments are overlapping for maximal interaction with myosin

154. A 34-year-old woman presented with pelvic pain, and ultrasound revealed a cystic ovarian mass. The multiloculated cyst pictured here was removed. The tumor can best be described as

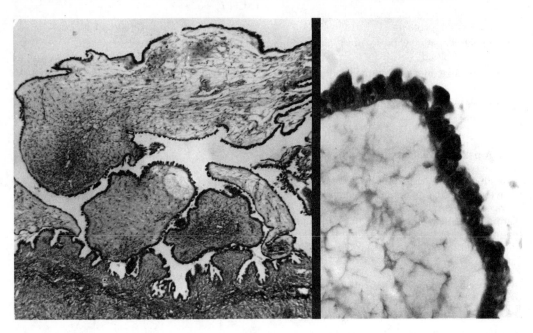

(A) being associated with elevated production of the beta subunit of human chorionic gonadotropin

(B) a germ cell tumor requiring interventional chemotherapy

(C) being rare outside of the elderly female population

(D) being an indolent low-grade neoplasm

Questions 155–157

A 48-year-old homeless man appears ataxic and confused in the emergency room. He is unshaven, mildly jaundiced, and has a bleeding scalp wound over the right frontotemporal area.

155. The physician should first

(A) ask the nurse to shower him, using antilice treatment

(B) suture his head wound

(C) order skull films

(D) obtain a serum ethanol level

(E) perform a neurologic examination

156. The patient suddenly falls into unconsciousness. The most emergent condition to assess would be

(A) subdural hematoma

(B) epidural hematoma

(C) delirium tremens

(D) hepatic encephalopathy

(E) AIDS

157. Appropriate treatment of delirium tremens includes all of the following EXCEPT

(A) monitor for generalized seizures

(B) treat with intravenous fluids

(C) monitor vital signs for autonomic arousal

(D) treat with chlordiazepoxide

(E) treat with disulfiram (Antabuse)

158. Which of the following pathophysiologic changes may be most useful in documenting, within less than 6 hours, that a patient had a myocardial infarction?

(A) Inverted or biphasic T wave on an electrocardiogram
(B) Elevated serum levels of creatine kinase
(C) Elevated serum levels of myocardial lactate dehydrogenase
(D) Maximal indices of coagulative necrosis
(E) Peak tissue infiltration of neutrophils

159. Which one of the following factors differentiates viruses from *Chlamydia*?

(A) Obligate intracellular parasitism
(B) The need for arthropod vectors
(C) Dependency on the host cell for energy
(D) The presence of a single type of nucleic acid

160. All of the following statements describe the genetic code EXCEPT

(A) it is nearly identical for all organisms
(B) it is composed of nucleotides containing three nucleotide code letters
(C) it represents all of the nucleotide sequence information within a transcription unit
(D) it contains transcription start and stop sequences
(E) it contains more than one codon for each amino acid

Questions 161–162

Five percent of individuals comprising a particular population are known to carry a recessive gene for poliodystrophy, an inherited disorder characterized by the onset of recurrent seizures and dementia in early childhood. A 32-year-old woman who had a brother with this disorder seeks genetic counseling. The patient's husband, an only child, does not know if his family has a history of the disorder.

161. What is the probability that the patient is a carrier of poliodystrophy?

(A) 1/20
(B) 1/10
(C) 3/8
(D) 2/3
(E) 3/4

162. What is the probability that both the patient and her husband are carriers?

(A) 1/30
(B) 1/20
(C) 3/8
(D) 2/3
(E) 3/4

Questions 163–164

The left ventricular and aortic pressure tracings below were recorded during cardiac catheterization of a 62-year-old patient who complains of chest pain and dizziness on exertion.

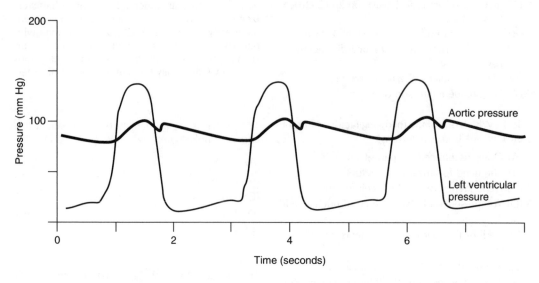

163. The left ventricular and aortic pressure tracings indicate that this patient has

(A) pulmonary stenosis
(B) aortic stenosis
(C) mitral stenosis
(D) aortic insufficiency
(E) mitral insufficiency

164. The most likely change in heart sound in this patient would be

(A) systolic murmur
(B) diastolic murmur
(C) presystolic murmur
(D) mid-diastolic murmur

---

165. All of the following enzymes may be targets of a new drug that inhibits cellular synthesis of DNA EXCEPT

(A) DNA-dependent DNA polymerase
(B) topoisomerase II
(C) RNA-dependent DNA polymerase
(D) RNA polymerase
(E) DNA ligase

166. Of the following cell types, which would contain many mitochondria in the apical portion of the cell?

(A) Smooth muscle cells
(B) Proximal convoluted tubule cells
(C) Steroid-secreting cells
(D) Liver parenchymal cells
(E) Skeletal muscle cells

167. Which of the following statements most accurately describes specific features of neuromuscular transmission?

(A) Each muscle fiber contains multiple axon terminals
(B) The end-plate is highly enriched in electrically excitable gates
(C) Enzymatic degradation of the transmitter can terminate transmission
(D) Acetylcholine (ACh) causes chloride channels to open as a result of membrane depolarization

168. A man acquires a "cold sore" from his girlfriend through ordinary kissing. Assuming this man will exhibit recurrent infections, which nerve axon might this disease traverse during reinfection?

(A) Cranial nerve (CN) VII (upper and lower buccal branches)

(B) CN V and the marginal mandibular branch of CN VII

(C) CN V_2 and CN V_3

(D) CN V_1 only

169. Chronic type B (antral) gastritis is characterized by all of the following features EXCEPT

(A) glandular atrophy with the presence of very few short, cystically dilated glands

(B) circulating antibodies to parietal cells and intrinsic factor

(C) excess acid secretion with low intragastric pH and, frequently, duodenal ulcers

(D) low serum gastrin levels

(E) flattened or absent rugal folds

170. The process of DNA replication can be best described by which of the following statements? DNA replication

(A) initiates at random sites on the chromosome

(B) of the *Escherichia coli* chromosome starts at multiple origins

(C) is unidirectional for all DNAs

(D) is not dependent on the synthesis of RNA primers

(E) occurs during the G_2 phase of the cell cycle

171. A 20-year-old man has a penile lesion that is crateriform, moist, and indurated. The patient revealed that this lesion has been present for about 20 days and is not painful. Which one of the following groups of tests is most appropriate?

(A) Gram stain, Venereal Disease Research Laboratory (VDRL) test, and culture of the lesion for *Treponema pallidum*

(B) Gram stain and culture of the lesion for *T. pallidum*

(C) VDRL and darkfield examination

(D) Fluorescent treponemal antibody absorption (FTA-ABS) test

172. Which one of the following techniques would be the best way to study a new kind of growth factor that induces proliferation of certain cell types?

(A) Measure uptake of radiolabeled methionine into cells after addition of the growth factor

(B) Measure uptake of radiolabeled thymidine into cells after addition of the growth factor

(C) Measure uptake of radiolabeled uracil into cells after addition of the growth factor

(D) Trypan blue exclusion

173. Which of the following areas of the central nervous system (CNS) contains structures that are considered to be phylogenically the oldest parts of the brain?

(A) Frontal lobe

(B) Limbic system

(C) Cerebellum

(D) Visual cortex

174. RNA processing can be best described by which of the following statements? It

(A) occurs in the cytoplasm

(B) results in the addition of nucleotides to the primary transcript of ribosomal RNA (rRNA)

(C) results in the formation of new covalent bonds between RNA and DNA

(D) includes the addition of a tail of polyadenylic acid at the 5' end

(E) includes the methylation of nucleotides in RNA

Questions 175–176

A research laboratory has been asked to study a new viral disease, which the researchers think is caused by an arenavirus. They need a relatively simple test to determine if this is indeed true. They have found a cell line (by pure chance) in which they can culture the virus.

175. The most specific trait of Arenaviridae that would help classify the new virus as a member of this family would be

(A) an insect vector

(B) the presence of multiple genomic segments

(C) the presence of particles resembling ribosomes within the virions

(D) the presence of a viral envelope

176. What is the best method to test for the presence of this trait?

(A) Gel electrophoresis; the gel is stained with ethidium bromide

(B) Grinding up a number of the presumed insect vectors, and preparing a filtrate of this material to infect cultured human cells

(C) Addition of virion fractions to radiolabeled amino acids, adenosine triphosphate (ATP), and human messenger RNA (mRNA); then detergent gel electrophoresis

(D) Light microscopy with a simple hematoxylin–eosin stain, with visualization of viral inclusion bodies

Questions 177–178

A 10-year-old girl is seen by her pediatrician for flu-like symptoms that were followed (weeks later) by a peculiar expanding skin rash (erythema chronicum migrans) and monarthritis arthritis (months later). Clinical laboratory findings include a positive titer against *Borrelia burgdorferi*.

177. A likely diagnosis for this child includes which one of the following diseases?

(A) Leptospirosis

(B) Lyme disease

(C) Rocky Mountain spotted fever

(D) Relapsing fever

(E) Yaws

178. Assuming a spirochete is the causative agent in this child's syndrome, appropriate pharmacotherapy may include which one of the following drugs?

(A) Rifampin

(B) Penicillin

(C) Chloroquine

(D) Pentamidine

(E) Praziquantel

179. The tumor pictured in the photomicrograph below arises from which one of the following types of cells?

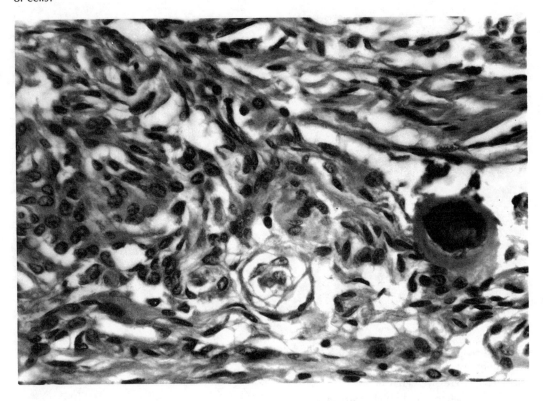

(A) Cerebellar astrocytes
(B) Leptomeningeal cells
(C) Neurons
(D) Oligodendrocytes
(E) Schwann cells

180. A 55-year-old man with a history of chronic alcoholism presents with complaints of fatigue and weakness. His laboratory values are as follows:

Hgb/Hct	11.5/34.0
MCV	110
MCH	38.0
RDW	19.5
WBC	$6.0 \times 10^9/L$

Differential:

Polys	80%	$4.8 \times 10^9/L$
Bands	7%	$0.42 \times 10^9/L$
Lymphs	10%	$0.6 \times 10^9/L$
Monos	5%	$0.3 \times 10^9/L$

Microscopic examination of a peripheral blood smear shows poikilocytosis and hypersegmented neutrophils. This patient most likely has

(A) anemia due to vitamin B deficiency
(B) anemia due to iron deficiency
(C) anemia following hemorrhage
(D) sickle cell anemia
(E) thalassemia minor

181. The hepatic neoplasm pictured below has which one of the following characteristics?

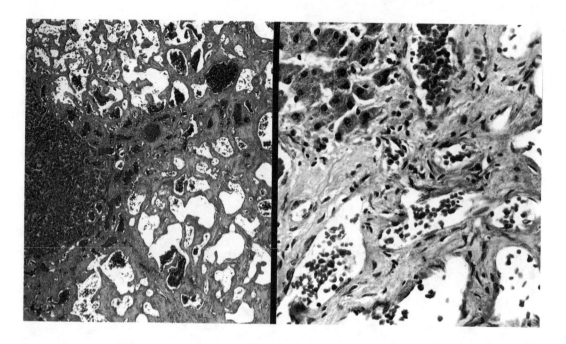

(A) An association with exposure to the carcinogen Thorotrast

(B) Highly aggressive behavior

(C) An association with thrombocytopenia

(D) Foci of hemorrhage and necrosis

182. All of the following thalamic nuclei are connected with the basal ganglia EXCEPT

(A) ventrolateral

(B) medial central

(C) pulvinar

(D) ventroanterior

183. The following sequence is a part of a globular protein. Which of the following statements best describes this peptide?

Ser-Val-Asp-Asp-Val-Phe-Ser-Glu-Val-Cys-His-Met-Arg

(A) At pH 7.4, the peptide has a net negative charge

(B) It has only one sulfur-containing amino acid

(C) The hydrophobic amino acid content exceeds the hydrophilic content

(D) Treatment with chymotrypsin would generate four smaller fragments

(E) Only three of the side chains are capable of forming hydrogen bonds

184. A rational approach for the treatment of ventricular tachycardia associated with myocardial ischemia in a hospitalized patient includes

(A) digitalis

(B) diltiazem

(C) lidocaine

(D) propranolol

(E) verapamil

185. What color would this tumor of the kidney (pictured) be?

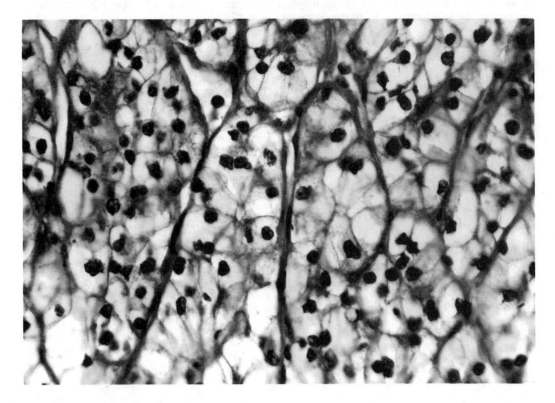

(A) Gray
(B) Translucent, with a pink hue
(C) White
(D) Yellow

186. If an individual has a genetic defect in the enzyme that produces *N*-acetylglutamate, the most likely clinical finding would be hyperammonemia with

(A) elevated levels of argininosuccinate (the condensation product of citrulline and aspartate)
(B) no detectable citrulline
(C) elevated levels of arginine
(D) elevated levels of urea
(E) no detectable ornithine

187. Which one of the following clinical procedures best demonstrates damage to the cerebellum?

(A) Testing for voluntary weakness by having the patient grasp the examiner's fingers and squeeze as hard as possible
(B) Tapping the patellar tendon and observing the reflex response
(C) Having the patient flex the neck, touching the chin to the sternum, to determine if this action elicits pain
(D) Passively moving the patient's limbs to elicit an increased resistance to motion

Directions: Each group of items in this section consists of lettered options followed by a set of numbered items. For each item, select the **one** lettered option that is most closely associated with it. Each lettered option may be selected once, more than once, or not at all.

Questions 188–191

For each organ listed below, select the region to which pain in that organ is usually referred.

(A) Inguinal and pubic regions
(B) Perineum, posterior thigh, and leg
(C) Both
(D) Neither

188. Ovary

189. Uterus

190. Epididymis

191. Testis

Questions 192–196

For each morphologic or functional description of a component of the placenta listed below, choose the appropriate lettered structure in the accompanying diagram.

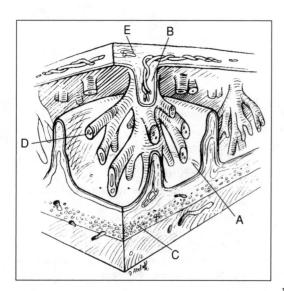

192. This structure is the decidual plate and is penetrated by maternal blood vessels

193. This structure is the intervillous space and contains maternal red blood cells

194. This structure is the chorionic plate and receives the insertion of the umbilical cord

195. This tissue column interconnects the chorionic and decidual plates

196. These structures are chorionic villi and are coated by syncytiotrophoblast

Questions 197–201

For each artery or vein comprising the vasculature of the cranium, select the lettered foramen or fissure through which it courses, shown on the illustration of the inferior aspect of the cranium below.

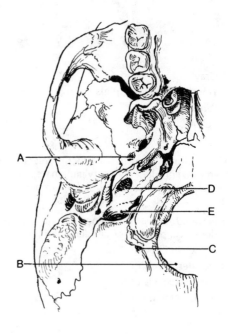

197. Middle meningeal artery

198. Internal carotid artery

199. Internal jugular vein

200. Emissary vein

201. Vertebral artery

Questions 202–206

Match each description involving thyroid hormones with the substance associated with it.

(A) Levothyroxine
(B) Thyrotropin-releasing hormone (TRH)
(C) Thyrotropin
(D) Iodine
(E) Thyroxine

202. In many forms of hyperthyroidism (Graves' disease), circulating levels of this hormone are considerably depressed

203. Propylthiouracil inhibits circulating levels of this hormone

204. This hormone is a L-pyroglutamyl-L-histidyl-L-proline amide whose intracellular signal transducing system involves phospholipase C activation

205. Deiodination of this hormone accounts for most of its ultimate biologic effects

206. A synthetic hormone useful for various forms of hypothyroidism

Questions 207–210

For each clinical state listed below, select the description of sleep architecture most closely associated with it.

(A) Sleep spindles
(B) Sleep-onset rapid eye movement (REM)
(C) Delta waves
(D) Increased percentage of REM
(E) Normal REM sleep

207. Narcolepsy

208. Major depression

209. Nocturnal penile tumescence

210. Night terrors

Questions 211–216

Lung tumors can at times have similar gross and microscopic appearances, but generally distinguishing features can be observed for the major tumor classes. Match the following descriptive features of malignant tumors with the correct neoplasm.

(A) Squamous cell carcinoma
(B) Adenocarcinoma (usual type)
(C) Adenocarcinoma (bronchioalveolar type)
(D) Large cell carcinoma
(E) Small cell (oat cell) carcinoma
(F) Carcinoid

211. Centrally located in major airways near the hilum; may have endobronchial element; large cells with optically dense cytoplasm form large irregular sheets with central necrosis; intercellular bridges; prominent host response; hypercalcemia

212. Grows along alveolar septa; multicentric foci; cuboidal or columnar cells with abundant mucus production; huge nuclei with almost no cytoplasm

213. Peripherally located; often associated with a preexisting scar; glandular, mucinous, or papillary growth pattern; prominent nucleoli; poorly differentiated tumors may be diagnosed by the presence of intracytoplasmic mucin

214. Often protrudes into the bronchus like a polyp; highly vascularized; small cells with monotonous round or fusiform nuclei; 80- to 250-nm neurosecretory granules; often grows in a pattern of clusters or ribbons of cells

215. Usually peripherally located; grows in sheets with areas of necrosis; small cells with scant cytoplasm and nucleoli that are not prominent; dense 80- to 140-nm neurosecretory granules; poor survival due to extensive metastases

216. Characterized by large nuclei, prominent nucleoli, and abundant cytoplasm; cells may be multinucleated; tumor displays well-defined cell borders; lack of mucin or keratinization often used for diagnosis

Questions 217–221

Match each description below with the appropriate organelle in the accompanying diagram.

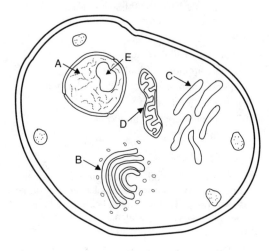

217. It is involved in the sorting and targeting of proteins

218. It is the site of cleavage of introns from messenger RNA (mRNA)

219. It is the site of ribosomal RNA (rRNA) synthesis

220. It is the site of steroid synthesis

221. It is the main site of adenosine triphosphate (ATP) synthesis

Questions 222–226

For each function, select the associated transport protein.

(A) Albumin
(B) Transferrin
(C) Haptoglobin
(D) Transcobalamin
(E) None of the above

222. Iron transport

223. Vitamin B_{12} transport

224. Clot formation

225. Plasma osmotic pressure maintenance

226. Hemoglobin transport

Questions 227–231

Match each clinical feature with the vitamin deficiency disorder or disorders most likely to be associated with it.

(A) Pellagra
(B) Beriberi
(C) Both
(D) Neither

227. Dermatitis

228. Peripheral neuropathy

229. Cardiovascular lesions

230. Dementia

231. Diarrhea

Questions 232–236

Match each of the following conditions with the appropriate syndrome.

(A) Sheehan's syndrome
(B) Cushing's syndrome
(C) Conn's syndrome
(D) Waterhouse-Friderichsen syndrome
(E) Bartter's syndrome

232. Hyperreninemia

233. Anterior pituitary infarction

234. An overproduction of cortisol

235. Widespread petechiae, purpura, or hemorrhages

236. Aldosterone-producing adenoma

Questions 237–240

Match each of the following descriptions with the appropriate segment or segments of the small intestine.

(A) Jejunum
(B) Ileum
(C) Both
(D) Neither

237. Contains well-developed plicae circulares

238. Contains many arterial arcades

239. May contain Meckel's diverticulum

240. Has appendices epiploicae on its external surface

Questions 241–244

Match each visual defect described below with the condition that causes it.

(A) Cataracts
(B) Astigmatism
(C) Presbyopia
(D) Myopia
(E) Hyperopia

241. A progressive decrease in the power of accommodation

242. A progressive loss of lens transparency

243. Focusing point of light rays is in front of the retina

244. Focusing point of light rays is behind the retina

Questions 245–248

A drug experiment was conducted, and the figures below show the results, which have been plotted in two different ways. Match each number in the figures with the most appropriate term.

(A) Maximal effect
(B) K_D
(C) $-1/K_D$
(D) $1/$Maximal effect
(E) None of the above

Questions 249–253

Match each of the following stages of mitosis with the appropriate term.

(A) Anaphase
(B) Early prophase
(C) Late prophase
(D) Telophase
(E) Metaphase

249. Dissolution of the nuclear envelope

250. Separation of the centromeres

251. First appearance of chromosomes

252. Alignment of chromosomes in the equatorial plane

253. Occurrence of cytokinesis

Questions 254–258

Match the pulse and pressure readings listed below with the most likely diagnosis.

(A) Normal
(B) Isolated systolic hypertension
(C) Autonomic neuropathy (e.g., diabetic neuropathy)
(D) Hypovolemia (dehydration)
(E) Hypertension

	Age	Sex	Pulse, supine	Blood pressure, supine	Pulse, sitting	Blood pressure, sitting
254.	74	F	60	140/80	65	128/85
255.	59	M	62	140/80	85	135/75
256.	68	M	72	138/76	74	124/63
257.	81	F	88	154/86	92	150/88
258.	63	M	64	145/92	66	147/94

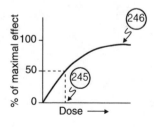

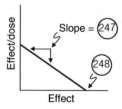

ANSWER KEY

1-D	31-A	61-D	91-C	121-C
2-A	32-C	62-B	92-C	122-A
3-C	33-C	63-D	93-B	123-D
4-A	34-C	64-A	94-B	124-A
5-B	35-B	65-B	95-C	125-E
6-C	36-D	66-A	96-D	126-A
7-A	37-D	67-D	97-C	127-B
8-D	38-A	68-C	98-D	128-C
9-E	39-E	69-A	99-A	129-D
10-B	40-C	70-D	100-D	130-D
11-E	41-A	71-C	101-D	131-B
12-B	42-A	72-C	102-A	132-C
13-B	43-D	73-D	103-B	133-E
14-D	44-C	74-E	104-D	134-A
15-C	45-B	75-C	105-B	135-B
16-C	46-A	76-D	106-D	136-D
17-A	47-C	77-D	107-E	137-D
18-C	48-E	78-B	108-E	138-D
19-C	49-E	79-A	109-A	139-C
20-C	50-A	80-A	110-C	140-E
21-A	51-D	81-B	111-B	141-C
22-C	52-C	82-D	112-C	142-C
23-D	53-C	83-C	113-B	143-C
24-D	54-B	84-A	114-E	144-C
25-A	55-A	85-D	115-D	145-C
26-D	56-C	86-D	116-C	146-C
27-C	57-D	87-B	117-A	147-D
28-A	58-C	88-C	118-E	148-A
29-B	59-E	89-D	119-D	149-E
30-B	60-A	90-D	120-B	150-D

151-B	173-B	195-B	217-B	238-B
152-C	174-E	196-D	218-A	239-B
153-A	175-C	197-A	219-E	240-D
154-D	176-C	198-D	220-C	241-C
155-E	177-B	199-E	221-D	242-A
156-B	178-B	200-C	222-B	243-D
157-E	179-B	201-B	223-D	244-E
158-A	180-A	202-C	224-E	245-B
159-D	181-C	203-E	225-A	246-E
160-C	182-C	204-B	226-C	247-A
161-D	183-A	205-E	227-A	248-C
162-A	184-C	206-A	228-B	249-C
163-B	185-D	207-B	229-B	250-A
164-A	186-B	208-D	230-A	251-B
165-C	187-B	209-E	231-A	252-E
166-B	188-A	210-C	232-E	253-D
167-C	189-C	211-A	233-A	254-A
168-C	190-B	212-C	234-B	255-D
169-B	191-A	213-B	235-D	256-C
170-E	192-C	214-F	236-C	257-B
171-C	193-A	215-E	237-A	258-E
172-B	194-E	216-D		

ANSWERS AND EXPLANATIONS

1. The answer is D. *(Pathology of Barrett's esophagus)*
Barrett's esophagus is a result of protracted reflux, due to lower esophageal sphincter incompetence, with the attendant increased exposure to acid, pepsin, and bile acids. Esophageal inflammation and ulceration occur, followed by re-epithelialization and ingrowth of immature pluripotent stem cells. Rather than squamous epithelium, the new epithelium is columnar-lined with gastric or duodenal-type cells, which better tolerate prolonged acid exposure. Inflammation would only be absent in the case of postmortem ulceration and autolysis; such changes may be accompanied by "leopard spotting" — brown–black esophageal spots that form from acid digestion of hemoglobin.

2. The answer is A. *(Plasma protein binding of drugs)*
Many drugs bind to plasma proteins, which limits glomerular filtration in the kidneys because the drugs are not freely diffusible. Drug protein interactions that are common generally occur between a wide variety of drugs and albumin or α_1-acid glycoprotein, but not immunoglobulins. Covalent interactions are rare, but when they occur it is generally with reactive antineoplastic drugs. Renal tubular secretion is generally not limited by plasma protein binding of drugs because secretion reduces free plasma drug concentration, which is quickly followed by dissociation of the drug from plasma proteins.

3–5. The answers are: 3-C, 4-A, 5-B. *(Suicide management)*
Safely removing any pill fragments from the stomach by nasogastric tube is the first step in the management of the patient described in the question because amitriptyline is an anticholinergic that retards gastrointestinal absorption, increasing the likelihood that pill fragments remain. The patient may ultimately need psychiatric hospitalization, but since she is unresponsive there is no urgency in pursuing this. An electroencephalogram would not add any useful information at this time, and seizures, if they occurred, would most likely be related to the toxicity of amitriptyline and a lowering of the seizure threshold.

Tricyclic antidepressants have antiarrhythmic effects, like quinidine. The changes on electrocardiogram, especially with increased or toxic serum levels, include a prolonged P-R interval, prolonged QRS duration, and a prolonged QT interval. In therapeutic dose ranges, tricyclics may suppress premature ventricular contraction.

Eliciting a detailed account of the events leading to the suicide attempt is important, particularly whether it was impulsive or well-planned or whether it occurred in the context of a depression. Once it has been established that suicide was in fact attempted, transfer to a psychiatric unit is imperative. In a crisis situation, the physician should avoid getting angry or overinvolved with the patient and should avoid prematurely interpreting underlying psychodynamic issues.

6. The answer is C. *(Membrane structure and function)*
The plasma membrane consists of amphipathic lipids (predominately phospholipids and cholesterol) and amphipathic proteins. The hydrophilic portions of these molecules face the external and internal aqueous environments. The hydrophobic portions are in the internal portion of the bilayer. Phospholipids prevent free diffusion of ions and water-soluble molecules, thereby imparting selective permeability properties to the lipid bilayer. Proteins may be restricted to the external portion of the bilayer or span it entirely. In addition, the membrane is fluid, allowing lateral diffusion of even large proteins.

7. The answer is A. *(Polymerase chain reaction)*
A polymerase chain reaction is used to amplify sequences of DNA from a single copy to over 1 million copies. The template DNA is initially denatured in the presence of excess primers, which are short (15–25 base pairs) oligonucleotides homologous to sequences on the template DNA. Because the DNA is denatured and renatured many times by multiple heating and cooling cycles, limiting amounts of primers prevents large-scale amplification of the parent strand. The temperatures at which a polymerase chain reaction is carried out are generally in the range from 55° C–95° C. Heat-resistant DNA polymerase, such as the Taq polymerase, is resistant to heat denaturation.

8. The answer is D. *(RNA structure and function)*
The primary transcript for messenger RNA (mRNA) is formed in the nucleus, where the elongation proceeds from the 5' to the 3' end. Most eukaryotic mRNAs are distinctive in that the 5' ends are capped by the addition of a methylated guanylic acid residue and the 3' ends have a polyadenylate tail of 100 to 200 adenosine nucleotides. Most precursor forms of mRNA contain intervening sequences, which are removed by a process known as splicing. The binding of steroid hormones with their receptors to specific genes results in the increased synthesis of the mRNA encoded in those genes.

9. The answer is E. *(Gastric carcinoma)*
Paget's disease of the breast is a carcinoma involving the nipple and subjacent ductal elements, and Paget's disease of the bone is an idiopathic disease characterized by a high turnover of bone. Neither form is associated with gastric carcinoma. The Leser-Trélat sign is the development of seborrheic keratosis, acanthosis nigricans, or amyloidosis in a patient with gastrointestinal malignancy. Erythema nodosum is seen occasionally with gastrointestinal malignancy.

BSGLC Basal Germinal Layer of Cornea

10. The answer is B. *(Epidermis)*
The order of epidermal maturation is stratum basale, stratum spinosum, stratum granulosum, stratum lucidum, and stratum corneum. The stratum basale is the germinal layer of the epidermis. Cells migrate and differentiate from this layer at a rate equal to desquamation of keratin from the outermost layer. The stratum spinosum is superficial to the stratum basale, and its cells are in the process of growth and early keratin synthesis. The stratum granulosum is characterized by the presence of intracellular granules, which contribute to the keratinization process. The stratum lucidum is a homogeneous layer between the stratum granulosum and the stratum corneum that is present only in thick skin. The stratum corneum is the most superficial layer of the epidermis and is mainly composed of keratin.

11. The answer is E. *(Recurrent urinary tract infections)*
Longitudinal studies have shown that bacteriuria in women susceptible to urinary tract infections is preceded by colonization of the vaginal introitus with the responsible organism from the rectal flora.

12. The answer is B. *(Gaucher's disease)*
Type II Gaucher's disease is the infantile acute cerebral pattern and is characterized by a virtual absence of glucocerebrosidase, with an accumulation of large quantities of β-glucosylceramide in macrophages and hepatocytes. Type I, or the classic form, is the adult type, in which storage of glucocerebrosides is limited to the mononuclear phagocytes. Patients with type I have reduced but detectable levels of glucocerebrosidase. Both type I and type II are autosomal recessive. Niemann-Pick disease is characterized by the accumulation of sphingomyelin, which is due to a deficiency in sphingomyelinase. Tay-Sachs disease, in which ganglioside accumulates, results from lack of N-acetylhexosaminidase. The defective enzyme in Krabbe's disease is galactosylceramidase.

13–15. The answers are: 13-B, 14-D, 15-C. *(Histology of the epididymis)*
The micrograph shows the epididymis. The epididymis is a highly convoluted tubular organ that conveys sperm and fluid from the testis to the ductus (vas) deferens. Its luminal epithelium is a pseudostratified columnar epithelium with numerous tall apical stereocilia. These cells secrete poorly characterized substances, which are added to the seminal fluid, and remove other poorly characterized substances from the fluids that drain from the seminiferous tubules in the testis. Apoptosis, or programmed cell death, occurs in the testis as in the thymus.

16. The answer is C. *(Pathophysiology of anthrax)*
A malignant pustule is a clinical manifestation of cutaneous anthrax. It occurs at the site of inoculation and is characterized by a black eschar at its base surrounded by an inflamed ring. Enteritis necroticans, caused by *Clostridium perfringens*, and pseudomembranous colitis, caused by *Clostridium difficile*, are diseases of the gastrointestinal tract that may be characterized by ulcerative lesions in the intestinal mucosa. Lockjaw is a lay name for tetanus; it refers to the muscle and neural spasms caused by the neurotoxin tetanospasmin. Woolsorter's disease is pulmonary anthrax — a diffuse, lethal, progressive pneumonia caused by the inhalation of spores of *Bacillus anthracis*.

17. The answer is A. *(Histopathology of seminomas)*
Seminomas comprise 30%–40% of testicular tumors and are divided into classical and spermatocytic forms. Classical seminomas, as in this case, are composed of nests of tumor cells with abundant clear cytoplasm with vesicular nuclei and angulated nucleoli *(left)*. The nests are separated by fibrous strands that contain inflammatory cells, usually lymphocytes and plasma cells *(right)*. Mumps orchitis involves large numbers of giant cells; it is an inflammatory reaction, not a neoplasm, and the condition is seen in young individuals. Teratomas contain aberrant ectopic tissues (e.g., brain, cartilage, and epithelial-lined cysts), while choriocarcinomas have syncytiotrophoblastic giant cells and cytotrophoblasts in close apposition.

18. The answer is C. *(Platelet homeostasis)*
Examination of the peripheral blood smear is essential when evaluating a patient for thrombocytopenia. Unreported abnormalities of the red cells may offer a clue to the etiology, or occasionally one may find

a discrepancy between the number of platelets seen on the smear and that found by the automated count. This occurs in pseudothrombocytopenia, where clumping of platelets in a specific anticoagulant [usually ethylenediaminetetraacetic acid (EDTA)] results in marked underestimation of the count.

19–21. The answers are: 19-C, 20-C, 21-A. *(Immunologic disorders)*
Patients with diseases that cause a deficiency in T cells are extremely prone to viral, fungal, and protozoal infections. The patient described in the question presents with severe oral thrush, which is caused by a *Candida* species, and hypocalcemia. These findings are consistent with a diagnosis of DiGeorge syndrome, which results from a defect in the embryonic development of the third and fourth pharyngeal pouches. Both the thymus and parathyroid glands fail to develop, resulting in hypocalcemia. The white blood cell count can be within normal limits, but virtually all of the circulating leukocytes are B cells and plasma cells.

DiGeorge syndrome does not appear to be genetically determined but occurs as the result of intrauterine damage. Without intervention, these patients have a poor prognosis. Transplantation of a fetal thymus not older than 14 weeks (to avoid graft-versus-host disease) has resulted in prolonged survival. Administration of antifungal agents will not really address the problem, which is a lack of T cells, and fungal infections may be a side effect of corticosteroid use.

Although both chronic mucocutaneous candidiasis and severe combined immunodeficiency result in increased susceptibility to viral, fungal, and protozoal infections, neither disease presents with hypocalcemia. Patients with chronic granulomatous disease, due to phagocytic cell dysfunction, suffer from infections with organisms that are normally of low virulence, such as *Staphylococcus epidermidis*, and also do not present with hypocalcemia.

22. The answer is C. *(Fluid balance)*
Infusion of a hypertonic solution instantaneously adds both volume and milliosmoles to the extracellular (and total body) water space. Because the solution is hypertonic, the osmolality increases in the extracellular space (but remains unchanged in the intracellular space), thereby causing osmosis of water out of the cells and into the extracellular compartment. At equilibrium, the extracellular volume is expanded, and its osmolality is increased. In contrast, the intracellular volume is decreased, resulting in an increase in intracellular osmolality.

23. The answer is D. *(Vaccines as applied to AIDS)*
Of the vaccination procedures listed, the one most likely to be tested by the Food and Drug Administration (FDA) is the procedure that uses a human monoclonal antibody that reacts with the intact CD4 (T4) receptor. Antibodies that react with CD4 should "look like" the portion of human immunodeficiency virus (HIV) that reacts with the CD4 receptor. Therefore, the vaccinated person should make an antibody to the human monoclonal antibody, which may be protective against HIV.

24. The answer is D. *(Immunologic response)*
The necessary characteristics that a given compound must possess to be immunogenic include a high molecular weight, chemical complexity, and recognition as being foreign. Compounds with a molecular weight greater than 6000 daltons are generally immunogenic, and those with a molecular weight less than 1000 daltons generally are not. Compounds between 1000 and 6000 daltons may or may not be immunogenic, depending upon the degree of foreignness or chemical complexity.

Haptens are small, low molecular weight compounds that become immunogenic when coupled to a high molecular weight carrier, such as a conjugate of dinitrophenol and albumin. While a large homopolymer of lysine would not be immunogenic because of a lack of chemical complexity, a smaller polymer containing different molecules would be immunogenic.

25. The answer is A. *(Glycolysis)*
The primary step in the regulation of glycolysis is the conversion of fructose 6-phosphate to fructose 1,6-bisphosphate. The enzyme, 1-phosphofructokinase, is an allosteric enzyme that is inhibited by adenosine triphosphate (ATP) and citrate and is activated by fructose 2,6-bisphosphate. The concentration of fructose 2,6-bisphosphate is, in turn, regulated by glucagon. Acetyl coenzyme A (acetyl CoA) is not an allosteric effector of any of the glycolytic enzymes. Glucose 6-phosphate is an inhibitor of hexokinase.

26. The answer is D. *(Renal sodium transport)*
Almost 75% of Na^+ is reabsorbed in the proximal tubular epithelium by several processes, including: active transport at the basolateral surface leading to electrogenic potential with additional passive movement; and cotransport of Na^+ at the luminal surface with glucose or amino acids. An additional 22% is

reabsorbed by the active transport process in the ascending thick limb of the loop of Henle. The remaining small percentage of Na^+ that reaches the distal tubular epithelium is reabsorbed by a highly regulated aldosterone-sensitive process involving exchange with K^+.

27. The answer is C. *(Papillary carcinoma)*
The photomicrograph is of a papillary carcinoma of the thyroid gland, and there is a demonstrated association of this type of tumor with previous radiation therapy to the neck. The tumor cells grow on thin fibrovascular stalks and form papillae. The cells have large overlapping nuclei; the nucleoplasm has marked chromatin, which gives the nuclei a clear, "Orphan Annie eye" appearance. Papillary carcinomas also may have stromal calcification, forming concentric laminated concretions called psammoma bodies *(top center)*. These carcinomas metastasize through the lymphatics to cervical lymph nodes, but, in general, they are very indolent tumors.

28. The answer is A. *(Pathogenic mechanisms of respiratory pathogens)*
Pertussis and diphtheria are caused by *Bordetella pertussis* and *Corynebacterium diphtheriae*, respectively. Both of these pathogens are extracellular bacteria, which adhere to the respiratory tract and produce exotoxins that contribute to pathogenesis. Since *B. pertussis* is gram-negative, it produces endotoxin, unlike gram-positive *C. diphtheriae.* The neurologic problems associated with the DTP (diphtheria-tetanus-pertussis) vaccine are due to the pertussis component of the vaccine (which uses whole killed cells).

29–31. The answers are: 29-B, 30-B, 31-A. *(Geriatric depression; pharmacologic migraine headache)*
The patient described in the question is suffering from depression. Monoamine oxidase inhibitor antidepressants (e.g., phenelzine) have a safe cardiac profile (except for some initial orthostatic hypotension) and essentially no anticholinergic activity, making them a good choice in the elderly who are vulnerable to constipation, memory impairment, and urinary retention. Lithium carbonate has a prophylactic role for recurrent depression but not acute depression. The neuroleptic chlorpromazine is not indicated because the patient is exhibiting no psychotic symptoms. Benzodiazepines (e.g., clonazepam) help with anxiety, which this patient does not have, and can sedate, increase cognitive deficits, and increase depression in the elderly.

A negative neurologic examination and lack of sleep disruption from the headache makes a brain tumor a less likely diagnosis. In elderly individuals, temporal arteritis is an important cause of head pain and blindness that necessitates prompt diagnosis and treatment with a corticosteroid. Computed tomography scan, cerebrospinal fluid examination, or an electroencephalogram would not aid in diagnosing temporal arteritis.

Lithium is useful for cluster headaches. Ergotamine may interrupt migraine headaches, while methysergide, propranolol, and amitriptyline have prophylactic value.

32. The answer is C. *(T-cell maturation)*
Maturation of a stem cell to a resting T cell occurs earliest in the cortex. The medullary region is where the variable (V), diverse (D), and joining (J) regions of the T-cell receptor undergo rearrangement. The maturation process is independent of antigen and dependent on contact with thymic epithelial cells for purposes of proliferation and differentiation.

33. The answer is C. *(Zellweger syndrome)*
In Zellweger syndrome, the amount of cytosolic catalase is elevated, phytanic acid accumulates in central nervous system (CNS) tissues, the plasma ratio of C26:0/C22:0 fatty acids is elevated, and there is a deficiency of platelet activating factor (PAF). Zellweger syndrome results from the absence of or a grossly reduced number of peroxisomes. Peroxisomes are cellular microbodies where oxidation of a very long chain of fatty acids (C26–C40) is initiated, phytanic acid is oxidized, and plasmalogens (such as PAF) are synthesized.

34. The answer is C. *(Gonorrheal and chlamydial coinfections)*
Of all cases presenting clinically as gonorrhea, 45% have coexisting chlamydial infections. Therefore, the correct treatment for gonorrhea is the administration of both penicillin for *Neisseria gonorrhoeae* and tetracycline for *Chlamydia trachomatis.* Amoxicillin is an oral penicillin; probenecid increases its blood level by blocking its excretion.

35. The answer is B. *(Mycology)*
Cryptococcus neoformans is responsible for meningitis in this case. The india ink microscopic staining technique demonstrated the presence of yeast cells producing a capsule (the capsule appears as a clear

halo), and the only encapsulated yeast among the options is *C. neoformans*. This organism is an important fungal cause of meningitis, and it often infects AIDS patients.

36. The answer is D. *(Pharmacologic action of aspirin and acetaminophen)*
Aspirin and acetaminophen are both effective antipyretic and analgesic drugs. However, acetaminophen is devoid of anti-inflammatory actions, whereas aspirin is the prototype of a group of nonsteroidal anti-inflammatory agents. Aspirin, but not acetaminophen, is associated with a risk of Reye's syndrome in pediatric patients treated for various viral diseases. Both aspirin and acetaminophen inhibit lipoxygenase activity.

37. The answer is D. *(Angiotensin-converting enzyme inhibitors)*
Captopril is the prototype of a group of angiotensin-converting enzyme (ACE) inhibitors. These agents lower blood pressure in poorly understood ways, but a critical role for inhibition of ACE (with loss of production of angiotensin II) seems apparent. ACE inhibitors do not affect renin per se, nor do they have any activity towards angiotensin II receptors.

38. The answer is A. *(Insulin-dependent diabetes mellitus type I therapy)*
Sulfonylureas and other oral hypoglycemics are contraindicated in insulin-dependent diabetes (IDDM). Insulin therapy to maintain blood glucose levels within a physiologic range is a symptomatic approach to the treatment of IDDM. Blood glucose levels are routinely monitored, and insulin is adjusted to maintain the blood glucose levels. A frequent side effect is hypoglycemia, which is best treated by ingestion of carbohydrates. Some patients who still maintain a normal response to glucagon benefit by injection of glucagon for this crisis as well. Although recombinant forms of insulin have reduced insulin insensitivity due to an immune response, this problem still persists. Apparently the source of the hormone (animal versus human) is not the only determinant of antigenicity.

39. The answer is E. *(Allosteric enzymes)*
Allosteric enzymes have sites distinct from the active site where regulatory ligands bind and alter either the V_{max} or the K_m for the substrate. The substrate saturation curves do not obey Michaelis-Menten kinetics and frequently show sigmoidicity, which is indicative of positive cooperativity between active sites. Enzymes that obey Michaelis-Menten kinetics require an 81-fold increase in substrate concentration to achieve an increase from 10% to 90% of the V_{max}. Allosteric enzymes that display positive cooperativity require a smaller increase in substrate concentration to achieve the same increase in V_{max}. The allosteric sites may be located either on the same subunit as the catalytic site or on a separate regulatory subunit. Enzymes with these regulatory properties frequently catalyze reactions that are either rate-limiting or occupy a pivotal point in a metabolic pathway.

40. The answer is C. *(Knee)*
The medial collateral ligament prevents abduction of the leg at the knee. It extends from the medial femoral epicondyle to the shaft of the tibia. The oblique popliteal ligament resists lateral rotation during the final degrees of extension. The posterior cruciate ligament prevents posterior displacement of the tibia. The anterior cruciate ligament helps lock the knee joint on full extension.

41. The answer is A. *(Female reproductive system)*
Blood flows to the fallopian tubes through branches of the uterine vessels carried in the surrounding mesentery, which is called the mesosalpinx. The ovarian veins drain blood from the ovaries. The right ovarian vein drains into the inferior vena cava; the left ovarian vein drains into the left renal vein. Lymph from the cervix eventually drains into the internal and external iliac and obturator nodes. Visceral afferent nerves from the uterus follow two pathways: Fibers from the cervix follow the splanchnic nerves (nervi erigentes); however, the body of the uterus and uterine tubes send fibers in parallel to the sympathetic nerves.

42. The answer is A. *(Histopathology of papilloma virus)*
This cervical tissue shows the squamous epithelial changes seen with human papilloma virus (HPV) infection, an epidemic affecting primarily young women. The viral infection causes crenation of nuclei and hyperconvolution, which is accompanied by perinuclear clearing of the cytoplasm. This change has been called condylomatous or koilocytic change and is due to HPV infection. Some subtypes of HPV predispose the cervical squamous epithelium to dysplasia, and, therefore, these patients are sometimes treated with ablative surgery.

43. The answer is D. *(Chemotherapy and biology of bacteria)*
Tetracycline inhibits protein synthesis in bacteria after it is selectively transported inside the cell by an active transport system. Tetracycline is selectively toxic not only because its transport system is peculiar to prokaryotes but also because it binds to 30S subunits of bacterial ribosomes. In bacteria (as well as in eukaryotic mitochondria), it prevents the binding of charged transfer RNA (tRNA) to the A site on the ribosomal complex, thereby inhibiting peptide bond synthesis. Thus, it is bacteriostatic, not bactericidal. Resistance can develop secondarily to altered influx or efflux of the drug in prokaryotes. It remains in the gastrointestinal tract and causes its most serious side effects there, either by direct irritation or secondary to modifications in gut flora. This can lead to life-threatening colitis. Tetracycline is hardly ever used in children because it accumulates in developing teeth and bones, causing stains and bone deformities.

44. The answer is C. *(Gluconeogenesis)*
Gluconeogenesis utilizes the enzymes in glycolysis that catalyze reversible reactions. The enzymes that catalyze irreversible steps in glycolysis are hexokinase, 1-phosphofructokinase, and pyruvate kinase. In order to circumvent the three irreversible reactions, the de novo synthesis of glucose requires four enzymes that are unique to gluconeogenesis: pyruvate carboxylase, phosphoenolpyruvate carboxykinase, fructose 2,6-bisphosphatase, and glucose 6-phosphatase.

45–47. The answers are: 45-B, 46-A, 47-C. *(Properties of anesthetic gases)*
Minimum alveolar concentration (MAC) is that concentration of anesthetic at 1 atm that produces immobility in 50% of patients exposed to a noxious stimulus.

If an anesthetic has a high blood:gas partition coefficient, it is very soluble in blood and is eliminated from the bloodstream into the alveolar air relatively slowly. This tends to prolong recovery time.

Relative potency of anesthetics is directly proportional to their lipid solubility. Among the commonly used agents, nitrous oxide has a very low oil:gas partition coefficient. In contrast, nitrous oxide has a rapid onset of action because of a low blood:gas partition coefficient. Nitrous oxide is neither explosive nor highly metabolized.

48. The answer is E. *(Dopamine receptor antagonism; tardive dyskinesia)*
Metoclopramide is a potent dopamine receptor antagonist that can cause tardive dyskinesia in nonpsychiatric patients. Tardive dyskinesia frequently involves the orobuccal area. Dystonia is a sustained muscle spasm that occurs as an early complication of treatment with an antidopaminergic drug. Wilson's and Huntington's diseases cause chorea, but there is no history to suggest these diseases.

49–54. The answers are: 49-E, 50-A, 51-D, 52-C, 53-C, 54-B. *(Pathophysiology and treatment of gout)*
Of the tests listed in the question, synovial fluid analysis, erythrocyte sedimentation rate, C-reactive protein, and differential white blood cell count may be useful in discriminating inflammatory versus noninflammatory musculoskeletal disorders. Synovial fluid analysis reveals clear liquid containing long, needle-shaped, negatively birefringent intracellular crystals (sodium urate). The presence of these crystals and their ingestion by macrophages are typical findings with gout.

Neurologic workup reveals slight dysarthria and incoordination. These symptoms are sequelae of an inherited X-linked partial deficiency of hypoxanthine–guanine phosphoribosyltransferase. This enzyme converts hypoxanthine to inosinic acid. Its deficiency increases purine synthesis, which contributes to the hyperuricemia of gout. Lesch-Nyhan victims are identifiable at birth and are mentally retarded. Osteoarthritis and calcium hydroxyapatite deposition disease afflict the elderly.

Colchicine is the anti-inflammatory drug of choice for gout. Allopurinol inhibits xanthine oxidase, the enzyme that converts hypoxanthine to xanthine, and xanthine to uric acid. Thus, allopurinol decreases urate production and is efficacious for the treatment of gout.

55. The answer is A. *(Embryology of the cardiovascular system)*
Both branches of the fourth aortic arch remain intact during fetal development. In adults, the left aortic arch forms the aortic arch, and the right aortic arch forms the proximal segment of the right subclavian artery. During development, the first and second aortic arches all but disappear. In adults, they form the maxillary, hyoid, and stapedial arteries. The third aortic arch forms the common carotid artery. The fifth aortic arch disappears. The sixth aortic arch forms the proximal segment of the right pulmonary artery and the ductus arteriosus.

56. The answer is C. *(Etiology of autoimmune disease)*
Forbidden clones provide a supply of cells that can recognize self-antigens and will serve as cells to stimulate both humoral and cell-mediated immune responses, leading to autoimmunity. B-cell deficiency — primarily a lack of circulating B cells — is a major cause of hypogammaglobulinemia. Type I hypersensitivity (anaphylactic hypersensitivity) is mediated by humoral antibodies, which result from a normal immune response to exogenous antigens. The deletion of forbidden clones leads to tolerance to autoantigens — the opposite of autoimmunity.

57. The answer is D. *(Empiric antibacterial therapy in an immunocompromised host)*
The most likely diagnosis explaining the patient's condition is septic shock secondary to bacteremia. Chemotherapy for cancer is a common cause of neutropenia with subsequent fever and infection. The risk is high when the white blood cell count is less than $500/\mu l$. In addition, cold, clammy skin is indicative of peripheral vascular shutdown. Lactic acid buildup will lead to metabolic acidosis and compensatory rapid breathing. Patients with neutropenic fever must be treated with double broad-spectrum antibacterial agents for gram-negative rods, including *Pseudomonas*. The combination of piperacillin, a broad-spectrum beta-lactam, and gentamicin, an aminoglycoside that has broad gram-negative activity, is a good choice. In addition, penicillin–aminoglycoside combinations may be synergistic because of the different mechanisms of action of these agents: Penicillins are cell wall synthesis inhibitors, and aminoglycosides inhibit protein synthesis. Single-agent therapy with gentamicin or amikacin would not be as effective for resistant organisms. Both chloramphenicol and gentamicin are protein synthesis inhibitors and would not be expected to work synergistically.

58–60. The answers are: 58-C, 59-E, 60-A. *(Medical ethics)*
If the physician's sole concern is not to harm the patient with unnecessary worry, the guiding principle is nonmaleficence. If her sole concern is to be able to benefit the patient with urography (which is impossible if the patient refuses because of concerns about the risks), the guiding principle is beneficence. Both are possible. Justice is irrelevant, and gratitude (e.g., for the patient's patronage) is, at most, marginally relevant.

If the physician decides to do what others of her profession do in like circumstances, she is acting without appeal to the independent ethical principles of beneficence and nonmaleficence. Depending on what the professional practice standard dictates, the disclosure decision might prove to be respectful of autonomy or strongly paternalistic, but the decision would still be guided by professional practice. Weak paternalism is entirely irrelevant because the patient is competent.

If the physician is guided by respect for the patient's preferences, she is acting with respect for her patient's autonomy. If the patient would want disclosure, it is possible that such disclosure could fail to benefit him or could even harm him, so neither beneficence nor maleficence is guiding the physician's thinking. Clearly, the basis for her thinking is independent of the usual practice of her profession.

61. The answer is D. *(Ultraviolet damage to DNA)*
Ultraviolet (UV) light causes cross-linking of thymidine base pairs in DNA and cross-links thymidine to cytosine (forming pyrimidine–pyrimidine dimers). In bacteria such as *Escherichia coli*, these lesions are repaired by a system of proteins called the SOS system, which includes the RecA protein, which is involved in the recombination of normal DNA and the repair of damaged DNA, and thus it would not be advantageous to decrease its activity. Also, it would be foolish to overlap the genes concerned, for one pyrimidine base pair could potentially impair all the genes involved. Removal of introns would also be disadvantageous, due to the fact that introns are thought to act as buffers of inactive DNA so that a mutation can occur without disrupting the gene. Genes produced with low thymidine content, however, may be less susceptible to damage by UV radiation because fewer pyrimidine base pairs would be involved.

62. The answer is B. *(Identification of neuroblastoma)*
Neuroblastomas arise from neural crest cells of the adrenal medulla. The tumors are usually large and soft, with red–gray cut surface. They may be calcified, with areas of hemorrhage and necrosis. The tumor cells have hyperchromatic nuclei and indistinct eosinophilic cytoplasm. The nuclei are arranged in a spoke-like pattern around a characteristic central mass of neuritic cell processes, called Homer-Wright pseudorosettes, as seen in the illustration. Like pheochromocytomas, neuroblastomas produce catecholamines, but, unlike pheochromocytomas, they do not cause systemic hypertension.

63–64. The answers are: 63-D, 64-A. *(Turner syndrome)*
The patient presented in the question is a classic example of a child with Turner syndrome (i.e., short stature, webbed neck, cubitus valgus), which is best diagnosed through chromosome analysis. The

genotype of this patient is most likely to be 45,X. None of the other tests listed in the question would contribute to the diagnosis of Turner syndrome.

Short stature is not a characteristic feature of Klinefelter syndrome. Klinefelter syndrome is best defined as male hypogonadism that occurs when there are two or more X chromosomes and one or more Y chromosomes; however, the genotype 46,XXY is the most common. Short stature is a major finding in the other conditions listed in the question.

65. The answer is B. *(Amino acid catabolism)*
The amount of alanine released from skeletal muscle is greater than the amount that can be accounted for in muscle protein. The catabolism of many amino acids in muscle involves the transamination of α-amino groups from amino acids to pyruvate, producing alanine. Thus, the carbon skeleton of much of the alanine released from muscle is derived from glucose via the glycolytic pathway.

66. The answer is A. *(Malaria)*
Of the major diseases with geographic relevance, malaria is one of the few that can be rapidly life-threatening. The other diseases listed (i.e., chronic Chagas disease, amebic dysentery, mucocutaneous leishmaniasis, and giardiasis) are either chronically debilitating or subpatent in nature. Amebic dysentery and giardiasis are not life-threatening conditions, and it is not necessary to determine the causative species for treatment of either. No effective treatment exists for chronic Chagas disease, so rapid diagnosis is not essential. While determination of the species of *Leishmania* is useful in distinguishing cutaneous and mucocutaneous leishmaniasis in terms of treatment, both are long-term infections and are not life-threatening.

67–68. The answers are: 67-D, 68-C. *(Volume of distribution; half-life of elimination)*
The volume of distribution (V_d) is approximately 10 L. V_d is defined as V_d = dose/Cp, where Cp is the plasma concentration at zero time. In this case, the Cp can be estimated easily because the log plasma concentration versus time plot is linear; it is approximately 100 μg/ml. Thus,

$$V_d = \frac{(20 \text{ mg/kg}) (50 \text{ kg})}{0.1 \text{ mg/ml}}$$
$$= 10,000 \text{ ml}$$
$$= 10 \text{ L}$$

The half-life of elimination of this drug is approximately 4 hours. The half-life of elimination can be determined graphically from the slope of the linear plot. First, note the time when a given concentration (e.g., 50 μg/ml) was detected (5 hours). Next, determine the time when half the original value (25 μg/ml) was detected (9 hours). Then, calculate the half-life of elimination: 9 − 5 = 4 hours.

69. The answer is A. *(Protein post-translational modifications)*
After proteins are synthesized (translated), many are glycosylated in the lumen of the endoplasmic reticulum and the Golgi complex. Oligosaccharides are attached to proteins by N-glycosylation of asparagine side chains or by O-glycosylation of serine and threonine side chains. The transfer of oligosaccharides is mediated by an activated lipid carrier, dolichol phosphate.

70. The answer is D. *(Properties of tricyclic antidepressants)*
Tricyclic antidepressants, such as imipramine, inhibit neuronal uptake of norepinephrine, serotonin, and other central nervous system (CNS) amines. Potentiation of local concentrations of these amines may underlie the ability of these agents to reverse symptoms of depression after chronic administration over several weeks. The parent and metabolite compounds of many of these drugs can directly or indirectly affect cardiac function (including α-adrenergic receptor blockade) and, thus, may cause orthostatic hypotension and cardiac dysrhythmias. Indeed, suicide with these agents is quite common, and the cause of death is related to cardiac toxicity. The drugs do not appear to affect dopamine receptors significantly in the concentrations used clinically. Some agents are more selective for serotonin uptake (e.g., fluoxetine, which is not a tricyclic) than for norepinephrine uptake (e.g., desipramine, which is a tricyclic).

71–72. The answers are: 71-C, 72-C. *(Medical genetics and cystic fibrosis)*
The frequency of the cystic fibrosis gene is 1/40, the square root of the incidence. Remembering the Hardy-Weinberg law, the gene frequency is equal to the square root of the incidence (q^2). If the incidence = q^2 = 1/1600, then the square root of the incidence, the gene frequency (q), = 1/40.

The proportion of normal siblings of individuals with cystic fibrosis who would be expected to be carriers is 2/3. Due to the recessive pattern of inheritance of cystic fibrosis, each offspring has a 1 in 4 chance of inheriting the disease. This leaves a chance that 2 of the 3 individuals will be heterozygotes, or carriers, for the cystic fibrosis gene. A simple punnet square will reveal that of the possible genotypes one can have in the offspring (of those individuals carrying a recessive disorder), 1 in 4 will have the double dose, or be homozygous for the recessive gene. Two individuals will have a single dose of the recessive gene and be carriers, and one will be normal. Since in cystic fibrosis the carriers are not clinically affected, there would be 3 normal individuals possible in the offspring. Two of those three will be carriers, hence the 2/3 proportion.

73. The answer is D. *(Transplant immunology; immunosuppressive agents)*
Rejection that occurs a few minutes to a few hours after transplantation is termed hyperacute rejection. It is the result of preformed circulating antibodies to the graft that were made as a result of previous transplantations, blood transfusions, or pregnancies. It usually transpires minutes after the donor kidney is anastomosed, although it can proceed over a period of a few days. The antibodies activate the complement system, with ensuing swelling, interstitial hemorrhage, and thrombotic occlusion followed by outright infarction of the kidney. The only therapy is removal of the transplanted tissue.

74. The answer is E. *(Defense mechanisms)*
Borderline patients tend to view things as extremes of black and white, with little ability to perceive the gray zones. In splitting, negative feelings are split off and attributed to one person (or thing), while positive feelings are attributed to another, without the realization that people have both good and bad features. Borderline patients may also project, deny, displace, and manipulate, but the example in the question is of splitting.

75. The answer is C. *(Regulation of arterial blood pressure)*
A rise in arterial pressure within the carotid sinus or an increase in pressure secondary to mechanical massage leads to activation of baroreceptors, which subsequently causes inhibition of the central vaso-constrictor center with activation of the central vagal center. The net short-term effect is a decrease in blood pressure, heart rate, and cardiac output. Ultimately, baroreceptors adapt to the stimulus and are unimportant in the long-term regulation of blood pressure. Clamping of the carotid arteries (in a vagoto-mized animal) will decrease baroreceptor firing and remove inhibitory pathways from the central nervous system (CNS), leading to increases in pressure and heart rate.

76. The answer is D. *(Properties of lidocaine)*
Local anesthetics block Na^+ channels and decrease conductance of Na^+, thereby inhibiting depolariza-tion and normal conduction of action potentials. Small, myelinated nerve fibers are most sensitive, and differential sensitivity explains preferential blockade for pain sensation as opposed to other sensory modalities. Lidocaine is highly lipid-soluble and may cause convulsions in the central nervous system (CNS) if sufficient amounts are delivered to the brain. By affecting Na^+ channels in cardiovascular tissue, dysrhythmia and decreased contractility may ensue. The ester anesthetics, such as procaine, are substrates for plasma cholinesterases, whereas lidocaine is more slowly metabolized in the liver. Local anesthetics such as lidocaine are often used in spinal anesthesia to produce more widespread blockage of neurotransmission.

77. The answer is D. *(Cytoskeleton)*
In muscle cells, actin and myosin filaments cause muscle contraction by a process known as the "sliding filament hypothesis." In nonmuscle cells, actin is involved with endocytosis, exocytosis, cell locomotion, and cytokinesis. The mitotic spindle is composed of the microtubule protein tubulin, not actin.

78. The answer is B. *(Mitochondria)*
Mitochondria are organelles unlike the others within the cell. They contain a ring of DNA that encodes for some of the proteins they require; the rest are encoded by the nuclear genes. Mitochondria also use a slightly altered genetic code than that used by other mammalian genes: Mitochondria have only 22 transfer RNA (tRNA) molecules (as opposed to 32 in the nucleus), so that 1 tRNA molecule must cover more codons. Some codons are also different (e.g., UGA, a termination codon normally, is a tryptophan codon to mitochondrial tRNA). Finally, genes encoding the proteins overlap one another, perhaps reflecting the fact that the genome is so small (16,500 base pairs).

79. The answer is A. *(Presentation of cutaneous erythema)*
The etiologic agent of erysipeloid is *Erysipelothrix rhusiopathiae,* a bacterium widely distributed in the environment. Human erysipeloid is clinically described as a slowly spreading cutaneous erythema. Cutaneous edema is characteristic, and the disease is very painful. Cutaneous diphtheria is characterized

by a necrotic lesion sometimes associated with insect bites; the bite apparently provides the break in the skin through which toxigenic *Corynebacterium diphtheriae* enters the tissue. Cutaneous nocardiosis is characterized by draining sinus tracts discharging purulent exudate-containing granules. Pontiac fever and listeriosis do not have cutaneous manifestations.

80. The answer is A. *(Gene duplications)*
There are as many as 100 to 1000 gene families that contain similar sequences. β-Tubulins and β-like globins are perfect examples of duplicated gene families. There are at least two nonfunctional regions in the human β-like globin gene cluster that have sequences similar to functional β-like genes. Analysis of their DNA sequences shows that they retain their intron/exon structure, but some sequence drift has resulted in sequences that block transcription or terminate protein translation. Some gene duplications, such as those for ribosomal and transfer RNA (rRNA and tRNA), along with genes coding for histones, are necessary to meet the demands of the cell for messenger RNA (mRNA) transcripts. Although there is no accepted model for duplication, it is thought to involve unequal crossover during meiosis.

81. The answer is B. *(Hardy-Weinberg law)*
The frequency of carriers of Tay-Sachs disease can be calculated from the Hardy-Weinberg law, in which the carrier frequency is equal to 2 pq: q is calculated by taking the square root of the incidence, which gives the frequency of the gene, 1 in 60, and p is equal to 1 − q, or 60/60 − 1/60, which gives 59/60. As can be seen here, in most cases of rare diseases, p becomes equal to 1, and the carrier frequency then becomes 2q, or 2 × 1/60, which gives a carrier frequency of 1/30.

82. The answer is D. *(Lipid biochemistry and arachidonic acid metabolism)*
Leukotrienes are compounds formed as the result of the action of lipoxygenase on arachidonic acid. Platelet activating factor (PAF) is an ether phospholipid. Eosinophil chemotactic factor (ECF) is a set of peptides that produces a chemotactic gradient to attract eosinophils. Thromboxanes (TXA_2), like prostaglandins, are synthesized through the action of cyclooxygenase, a reaction that is inhibited by acetylsalicylic acid.

83–84. The answers are: 83-C, 84-A. *(Hypoxic injury)*
The first of the motor functions to become deficient during hypoxic injury to the brain would be the ability to move the arms. This is due to the fact that the most distal ends of the anterior and middle cerebral arteries anastomose in the cerebral hemispheres over the location on the motor gyrus controlling the arms. The neurons in this anastomosing zone are very sensitive to hypoxic injury.

The hippocampus is well-known for its sensitivity to hypoxic injury. Since this area of the brain is involved in immediate memory recall, the patient will not remember where he is nor will he remember his physicians. He will have trouble in the future functioning independently due to this lesion. Recognition of family members would involve distant, or remote, memory, which is not involved with hippocampal functioning. The patient would also be able to perform cognitive functions, such as addition and reading.

85. The answer is D. *(Surgical prophylactic antibacterial therapy; drug resistance)*
Ampicillin is an extended-spectrum penicillin, which has greater action against some gram-negative organisms compared to penicillin G and early generation semisynthetic penicillins such as methicillin. However, ampicillin is susceptible to beta-lactamases and may not be effective when administered prophylactically against beta-lactamase–containing *Staphylococcus aureus*. Cefazolin is a prototypical first-generation cephalosporin, which has good activity against staphylococcal infections and is relatively impervious to beta-lactamases. Methicillin is prototypical of beta-lactamase–resistant penicillins. Vancomycin is a cell wall synthesis inhibitor with exclusive gram-positive antibacterial activity, owing to its large molecular size, which does not allow it to enter gram-negative bacteria through porins. Vancomycin is not susceptible to beta-lactamases. Imipenem is a beta-lactam antibiotic, which is resistant to beta-lactamases.

86. The answer is D. *(Hypersensitivity reactions)*
ABO or Rh incompatibility, the cause of erythroblastosis fetalis, is the result of blood group differences between the mother and the child. Normally in cases of Rh-incompatible mating, human anti-D globulin (RhoGAM), an anti-Rh antibody, would be given to the mother shortly after the birth of her first Rh-positive child. This would clear the child's Rh-positive red cells from the mother's circulation before she can be immunized. In the case described in the question, the mother has blood type O negative with normal isohemagglutinin titers, so the preexisting ABO compatibility should clear her system of any "leaked" fetal blood cells. Administration of RhoGAM to an Rh-positive child will cause hemolytic anemia in that child.

87. The answer is B. *(Gas exchange)*
Anemia reduces the oxygen-carrying capacity of the blood but does not affect arterial oxygen tension. Thus, oxygen delivery is decreased and venous oxygen will have a lower partial pressure at rest and during exercise in the anemic subject. The anemic subject is patient *B* since his oxygen content is reduced for every level of Po_2.

88. The answer is C. *(Toxins; neurotransmission)*
The woman is suffering from botulism, which is caused by the neurotoxin botulin. The action of botulin involves inhibition of acetylcholine (ACh) release from peripheral nerve endings at the neuromuscular junction. Other bacterial toxins have actions described in (A), (B), (D), and (E) [i.e., diphtheria toxin, tetanus toxin, cholera toxin, and streptolysin O, respectively].

89. The answer is D. *(Gonococcal salpingitis)*
For all practical purposes, the patient is cured. However, women who suffered from gonorrhea are a population at risk for future complications, such as subsequent episodes of pelvic inflammatory disease, infertility, and ectopic pregnancy.

90. The answer is D. *(Hassall's corpuscles)*
Hassall's (thymic) corpuscles are found in the thymus. They are concentrically laminated structures of unknown function that appear during fetal development and increase in number with age. They are thought to be degenerated medullary epithelial cells and display varying degrees of keratinization or calcification.

91. The answer is C. *(Fructosuria; glycogen synthesis)*
Essential fructosuria results from a deficiency in fructokinase, which is found only in the liver and catalyzes the first step in the assimilation of fructose by the liver. Under normal conditions, almost all of the fructose is converted to fructose 1-phosphate and is metabolized in the liver. Hexokinase, which is present in all extrahepatic tissues, can convert fructose to fructose 6-phosphate; however, the K_m of hexokinase for fructose is sufficiently high that this reaction does not occur to any significant extent. When, as a consequence of a deficiency in fructokinase, the accumulation of fructose is high enough, it is converted to fructose 6-phosphate in extrahepatic tissues and metabolized by the glycolytic pathway. Glucokinase, which is found in the liver, is specific for glucose and cannot catalyze the phosphorylation of fructose. Aldolase B is specific for fructose 1-phosphate. Transketolase is a part of the nonoxidative phase of the pentose phosphate pathway.

92. The answer is C. *(Pathogenesis of renal osteodystrophy)*
Normally, approximately 90% of serum phosphate is not protein-bound and, thus, is filterable at the glomerulus. Of the filtered phosphate, about 75% is actively reabsorbed, mainly by cotransport with sodium in the proximal tubule. In chronic renal failure, hyperphosphatemia occurs as the glomerular filtration rate declines. Hyperphosphatemia produces a secondary hyperparathyroidism as excess phosphate ties up the free serum calcium, in essence leading to hypocalcemia. 1,25-Dihydroxyvitamin D_3 levels are reduced directly by the inability of the damaged kidney to convert the 25-hydroxyvitamin D_3 produced by the liver from inactive vitamin D_3 to 1,25-dihydroxyvitamin D_3 and indirectly by the ability of high serum phosphate levels to directly inhibit renal 25-hydroxyvitamin D_3 hydroxylase activity.

93. The answer is B. *(Differential diagnosis of coagulation disorders)*
Factor XI deficiency is autosomally transmitted and can result in serious postoperative bleeding, even though it may be mild enough to cause no spontaneous symptoms. Neither factor XII nor Fletcher factor deficiencies result in a bleeding disorder, and inherited factor VIII deficiency occurs only in males. Severe von Willebrand's disease could result in a positive family history and significant bleeding, but rarely is the factor VIII:C low enough to prolong the partial thromboplastin time (PTT), especially when the bleeding time is normal.

94. The answer is B. *(Enteric infections)*
Salmonella typhi is a highly invasive pathogen that is readily disseminated throughout the body. In typhoid fever, this organism invades through the intestinal mucosa and spreads through the body via the lymphatic system. In nontyphoid *Salmonella* infections, the bacteria invade into the intestinal submucosa but usually do not spread into other regions of the body. *Campylobacter jejuni* and *Shigella dysenteriae* invade the intestinal mucosa but usually do not penetrate the submucosa or spread throughout the body. *Vibrio cholerae* is noninvasive.

95–96. The answers are: 95-C, 96-D. *(Etiology of fungal infections; antifungal therapy)*
The clinical signs and history are consistent with oropharyngeal candidiasis (thrush). This patient is most likely immunocompromised due to her adjuvant chemotherapy. In addition, antibacterial therapy for urinary tract infection predisposes her to develop a fungal infection due to depletion of floral bacteria. Opportunistic, endogenous *Candida* infections in the mouth are common under these conditions. Sporotrichosis is an endogenous systemic infection. Cryptococcosis is also a systemic infection. Dermatophytes usually appear on hair, nails, and skin.

Griseofulvin is effective for dermatophyte infections of nails and hair; it concentrates in the stratum corneum and outer epidermis and stops fungal growth in these tissues. Ketoconazole, fluconazole, and clotrimazole are ergosterol synthesis inhibitors, which are fungistatic or fungicidal (at high concentrations) for *Candida*. Nystatin, a polyene, binds to membrane ergosterol and affects membrane permeability and integrity. Nystatin, like the more commonly used polyene amphotericin B, is fungicidal. Nystatin is effective only in topical preparations for candidiasis, whereas amphotericin B is commonly used systemically. Clotrimazole is effective topically against candidiasis.

97. The answer is C. *(Histopathology of rheumatoid arthritis)*
The synovium pictured in the photomicrograph shows the classic features of a rheumatoid nodule in a patient with rheumatoid arthritis, a disease that affects primarily women. Rheumatoid arthritis initially affects the small joints of the hands and feet and then the larger joints of the knees and elbows. The synovium becomes infiltrated by lymphocytes and plasma cells with lymphoid follicle formation. In some cases, central fibrinoid necrosis occurs with an intense palisade of histiocytes and giant cells forming around the necrotic material, as in this case. Rheumatoid nodules occur in the skin and subcutis, particularly on extensor surfaces, but may also occur in unusual sites as in the lungs, heart, and spleen.

98. The answer is D. *(Macroscopic features of Crohn's disease)*
The photomicrograph shows chronic inflammation of the bowel, typical of Crohn's disease, or terminal ileitis. This transmural inflammation accounts for the thickened bowel wall. If the process extends into pericolic fat, thick, edematous "creeping fat" and fistulae would be seen. The presence of a small granuloma at the base of the colonic gland is helpful in confirming the diagnosis of Crohn's disease. Pseudopolyps occur in ulcerative colitis and are a means of differentiating ulcerative colitis from Crohn's disease.

99. The answer is A. *(Functions of nucleic acids)*
RNA differs from DNA by the number of hydroxyl groups present on the sugar moieties and in the kind of pyrimidine bases used; RNA has uracil substituted for thymidine. Because these differences are fairly minor, RNA can take on the same configurations as DNA; that is, it can be linear, circular, double-stranded, or single-stranded. Molecules of transfer RNA (tRNA) are a perfect example of RNA that has base-paired with itself to form double strands. RNA acts catalytically in certain messenger RNA (mRNA) splicing reactions and is the primary genetic material for a number of viruses.

100. The answer is D. *(Histamine receptor antagonists)*
Cimetidine and ranitidine are H_2-receptor blockers whose main clinical use is in the treatment of ulcers and other peptic disorders. They block the effects of histamine on gastric acid secretion. H_2 antagonists inhibit, not enhance, cytochrome P450 enzymes of the liver. H_1 antagonists (diphenhydramine, chlorpheniramine, and so forth) are useful in treating allergies. They also have central effects that are useful in preventing motion sickness; however, they can also cause unwanted sedation.

101. The answer is D. *(Peptide bonds)*
The chemistry of the peptide bond imposes restrictions on higher orders of protein structure. The secondary structure of proteins is stabilized by hydrogen bonds that are formed between the amide hydrogen and carbonyl oxygen of the peptide bond. Because the atoms of the peptide bond lie in a plane, the only rotations that are permissible are around the $C\alpha$—C and the N—$C\alpha$ bonds. There is no formal charge associated with the peptide bond; the electrons of the carbonyl oxygen and the lone pair of electrons on the nitrogen atom are delocalized.

102. The answer is A. *(Calcium homeostasis)*
Ethylenediaminetetraacetic acid (EDTA) is a chelator of Ca^{2+} but is not normally found within cells and, thus, is not a mechanism by which cells regulate Ca^{2+} concentration. Two important transmembrane proteins in Ca^{2+} homeostasis are the Ca^{2+} adenosine triphosphatase (ATPase) pump and the Na^+–Ca^{2+} transport chain. Ca^{2+} binds to a number of intracellular proteins, such as calsequestrin, and these proteins are found in high concentration in the endoplasmic reticulum.

103. The answer is B. *(Medical genetics)*
Every child has a 50% chance of inheriting a condition with an autosomal dominant mode of inheritance. This does not mean that in a family with eight children, four will necessarily be affected and four unaffected, although this is statistically the most likely possibility. It is also possible that all children will be affected or all will be unaffected, although these possibilities are unlikely.

104. The answer is D. *(Enzyme inhibition)*
The data in the Lineweaver-Burk plot are diagnostic of noncompetitive inhibition. The intercept on the $1/[S]$ axis indicates that the inhibitor has no effect on the K_m for the substrate. The increase in the $1/v$ intercept observed in the presence of the inhibitor indicates a decrease in the V_{max} of the reaction. Noncompetitive inhibitors interact at a site other than the active site. They usually bear no structural resemblance to either the substrate or the transition-state analogs, and their effects cannot be reversed by high concentrations of substrates. Competitive inhibitors, however, interact at the active site, are structurally related to transition-state analogs, and can be reversed by high concentrations of substrate.

105. The answer is B. *(Serine and threonine kinases)*
Protein kinase C is a member of a class of kinases that phosphorylates only serine and threonine, not tyrosines. Protein kinase C is activated by lipids and Ca^{2+}; when activation occurs, protein kinase C moves from the cytoplasm to the plasma membrane via the process called translocation. It is degraded by a calcium-activated protease to form the Ca^{2+}- and lipid-independent protein kinase M.

106. The answer is D. *(Alveolar ventilation)*
Alveolar ventilation is the product of respiratory rate × (tidal volume − dead space). In this situation total dead space (400 ml) is the sum of the patient's anatomic dead space (150 ml) and the ventilator's dead space (250 ml). Thus, if the total output of the ventilator is adjusted to 600 ml, then 200 ml of the alveolar volume will be delivered 20 times per minute, and total minute alveolar ventilation will be 4 L/ min.

107. The answer is E. *(Microcirculation)*
Fenestrated capillaries have circular pores (fenestrae), which are 60 nm to 100 nm in diameter and may be partially surrounded by pericytes. The fenestrae often are spanned by a slit diaphragm, which is filamentous and, thus, does not possess a unit membrane structure. Fenestrated capillaries are present in areas where there is a great deal of molecular exchange with blood (e.g., kidneys, small intestine, endocrine glands, choroid plexus). Although glomerular capillaries are fenestrated, they lack a slit diaphragm; a thick basement membrane forms the filtration barrier.

108. The answer is E. *(Pathogenesis of infectious microorganisms)*
Borrelia burgdorferi is spread by ticks and is the cause of Lyme disease. *Rickettsia rickettsii* also is usually spread by ticks. *Clostridium tetani* enters the body through wounds. *Neisseria meningitidis* and *Corynebacterium diphtheriae* both enter via the respiratory tract.

109–111. The answers are: 109-A, 110-C, 111-B. *(Neurologic lesions and syndromes)*
The deficits described in the question indicate destruction of cranial nerve (CN) III motor function and total autonomic function of the eye, combined with a spastic paralysis of the contralateral body, indicating upper motor neuron destruction (as opposed to flaccid paralysis, indicating lower motor neuron disease). CN III fibers leave the brain at the level of the midbrain to continue to the ipsilateral eye. CN III is responsible for moving the eye nasally and vertically in both directions; hence, loss of CN III function results in lateral deviation of the eye. CN III also carries autonomic fibers that originate in the Edinger-Westphal nucleus and are responsible for constriction of the pupil to light and for accommodation. Riding with the oculomotor nerve are sympathetic fibers responsible for dilation of the pupil. The destruction of all of these functions together indicates a lesion of the midbrain where it intersects with the corticospinal tract.
  The artery that supplies this intersection of midbrain and corticospinal tract is the posterior cerebral artery. The basilar artery supplies the pons. The middle cerebral artery supplies most of the cerebral hemisphere of either side.
  Weber's syndrome is a lesion of the crus cerebri, through which the corticospinal tract passes, as well as a lesion of tissue through which the oculomotor nerve passes. Millard-Gubler syndrome is similar to Weber's syndrome, but the lesion is lower and involves the pons, causing CN VI and CN VII palsy as well as upper motor neuron paralysis of the contralateral body. Brown-Séquard syndrome is a lesion of the spinal cord, involving upper motor neuron damage and weakness of one leg, with contralateral pain and temperature sensitivity of the other.

112. The answer is C. *(Signal transduction; protein kinases)*
Protein kinase C is activated by Ca^{2+} and diacylglycerol, not by cyclic adenosine monophosphate (cAMP). Cyclic AMP is synthesized from adenosine triphosphate (ATP) in a reaction that is catalyzed by adenylate cyclase. The activity of adenylate cyclase may either be increased or decreased in response to hormone stimulation. Cyclic AMP is the second messenger for the effect of parathyroid hormone (PTH) on the kidney; cAMP also activates protein kinase A. The binding of cAMP to the regulatory subunit results in the dissociation of the regulatory and catalytic subunits and a concomitant increase in protein kinase activity. The degradation of cAMP is mediated by a family of phosphodiesterases, which catalyze the hydrolysis to 5'-AMP.

113. The answer is B. *(Glycogen storage diseases)*
Glycogen storage disease type Ia, or von Gierke's disease, is caused by defective glucose-6-phosphatase activity and is characterized by hepatomegaly, renomegaly, and hypoglycemia. The liver shows intracytoplasmic accumulation of glycogen and a small amount of lipid along with some intranuclear glycogen. The kidney has intracytoplasmic accumulations of glycogen in the cortical tubular epithelial cells. The intestine also shows increased concentrations of glycogen.

114. The answer is E. *(Tay-Sachs disease)*
Tay-Sachs disease has a reported 1 in 30 carrier rate among Ashkenazi Jews, which is about 10 times higher than in other population groups. It is a lysosomal storage disease caused by mutations in the gene coding for hexosaminidase A, leading to a virtual absence of this enzyme. Deficiency of hexosaminidase A results in an accumulation of GM_2 gangliosides, which normally make up 1%–3% of total brain gangliosides but comprise over 90% in individuals with Tay-Sachs disease. Lack of the enzyme β-galactosidase is an autosomal recessive disorder; however, unlike Tay-Sachs disease, it results in lysosomal storage of GM_1 gangliosides.

115–118. The answers are: 115-D, 116-C, 117-A, 118-E. *(Pathophysiology and pharmacotherapy of ischemic heart disease)*
Coronary blood flow closely matches myocardial work (or oxygen consumption). Myocardial oxygen extraction is near maximal at rest and does not increase appreciably, even during exercise. Coronary blood flow is maximal during diastole, in which ventricular compression of the capillaries is minimal. In addition, there is significant heterogeneity across the ventricular wall during systole, such that subendocardial blood flow is reduced, and blood flow is shifted to the epicardial vessels. Autoregulation is normally observed in the myocardium, such that blood flow does not change over a large range of perfusion pressures.

Nitroglycerin is metabolized to nitrosothiols that are similar or identical to the endogenous endothelial-derived relaxing factor, or nitric oxide. This metabolic product of L-arginine is synthesized in the endothelium (and other cells) and diffuses to smooth muscle cells, where it activates guanylate cyclase and induces relaxation.

The most significant adverse effect of nitroglycerin is unwanted systemic hypotension. This results in a reflex tachycardia due to decreased pressure that is sensed in peripheral baroreceptors.

A β-adrenergic receptor blocker (e.g., propranolol) is useful concomitant therapy with nitroglycerin, since it antagonizes the reflex tachycardia at the level of myocardial receptors.

119. The answer is D. *(Membrane physiology and excitation)*
The resting membrane potential is -90 mV, which is primarily due to diffusion potentials caused by K^+ (and Na^+) and the electrogenic Na^+–K^+ pump. Stimulation at time zero [e.g., as occurs with acetylcholine (ACh)] activates a Na^+ channel, thereby greatly increasing Na^+ conductance and leading to depolarization. At the peak of the action potential, the number of open Na^+ channels is 10 times greater than the number of open K^+ channels. Within a short period of time, voltage-gated Na^+ is inactivated, and a K^+ channel opens, greatly increasing the conductance to K^+ and, hence, repolarization. The Ca^{2+}–Na^+ channel (if present) is slow to be activated and normally would depolarize the membrane. Chloride channel permeability does not change during an action potential and, thus, functions passively in this process.

120. The answer is B. *(Neurologic disease)*
The patient described in the question most likely has tabes dorsalis, a disease that results from an untreated syphilis infection. The causative agent is *Treponema pallidum*, and the antibiotic of choice is penicillin. This disease results in the selective destruction of neurons in the spinal cord near the dorsal

root of the spinal nerves, which causes the symptoms described in the question. Varicella zoster virus (VZV) causes shingles, a disease resulting from the activation of the virus in dorsal root ganglia of the spinal nerves, and chickenpox, a vesicular disease that usually affects children. Acyclovir is an antiviral agent that interferes with VZV as well as herpes simplex virus replication and, hence, is not useful here.

121. The answer is C. *(Glomerular filtration rate)*
Blood enters the glomerulus via an afferent arteriole and leaves via an efferent arteriole. A decrease in renal blood flow (RBF) or a decrease in glomerular hydrostatic pressure tends to decrease the glomerular filtration rate (GFR). Accordingly, constriction of the afferent arteriole generally has this effect. An increase in RBF that increases hydrostatic pressure increases GFR. This effect of RBF persists even without an increase in hydrostatic pressure because of a subtle oncotic effect. Although raising systemic pressure would theoretically increase hydrostatic pressure and GFR, the effect is greatly minimized by normal autoregulation in the kidney. Thus, RBF and hydrostatic pressure is maintained by afferent arteriolar constriction in the presence of this increase over normal systemic pressures. Constriction of the efferent arteriole increases hydrostatic pressure (and GFR), but this effect is also offset by the above-mentioned decrease in RBF and, thus, only a modest increase in GFR is normally observed.

122. The answer is A. *(Neutropenia and infection)*
Neutropenia is defined as an absolute neutrophil count of less than $1500/\mu l$. While there is a modest risk of acquired infection beginning at this level, patients with neutrophil counts of less than $1000/\mu l$ for any length of time are at significant risk of acquired infection and patients with counts below $500/\mu l$ are at extreme risk. The percentages of formed elements determined by peripheral blood count are of limited value; they must be multiplied by the total white cell count to arrive at absolute numbers of circulating granulocytes, monocytes, and lymphocytes. Leukocyte percentages determined by a 100-cell manual differential count have extremely broad 95% confidence intervals that may yield broad apparent shifts in absolute numbers. New cell counters with machine analysis of percentages of neutrophils, monocytes, and lymphocytes (even eosinophils and basophils) offer a better estimate of absolute number.

123. The answer is D. *(DNA and RNA composition)*
DNA is composed of the purines adenine and guanine and the pyrimidines thymine and cytosine. RNA is composed of the same bases with the exception that thymine is replaced by uracil. Therefore, DNA or RNA can be selectively labeled by using tritiated thymine [(^{3}H)-thymine] or tritiated uracil [(^{3}H)-uracil], respectively.

124. The answer is A. *(Integral membrane proteins)*
Integral membrane proteins are stabilized by hydrophobic interactions between the lipid bilayer and the amino acid side chains. Detergents are required for solubilization. Approximately 20 amino acids in an α-helical conformation are required to span the width of the bilayer. These proteins display compositional asymmetry, with the carbohydrate moieties always being on the side of the membrane away from the cytoplasm. They may display lateral, but not transverse, movement within the membrane.

125. The answer is E. *(Urinary tract infection therapy)*
Penicillin G is the treatment of choice. It is inexpensive, and it is a broad-spectrum antibiotic effective in the treatment of urinary tract infections. The serum levels are so low that it is unlikely to alter the natural bacterial flora of the host.

126. The answer is A. *(Immunity to infection)*
Opsonic antibodies are important for acquiring immunity to infection by group A *Neisseria meningitidis* because they permit recognition and destruction of *N. meningitidis* at the onset of infection. *Vibrio cholerae, Clostridium botulinum,* and *Shigella flexneri* exert their pathogenic effects via toxins. Opsonic antibodies are not known to protect against the action of *V. cholerae, C. botulinum,* or *S. flexneri*.

127. The answer is B. *(Mechanics of the heart)*
At the end of the period of isovolumic contraction (*2*), the pressure inside the ventricle has risen to equal the pressure in the aorta at end diastole (80 mm Hg). At this point, ventricular pressures push the aortic valve open, and blood begins to pour out of the left ventricle (*3*) while it continues to contract. The fraction of end diastolic volume (115 ml) that was ejected was 60% since stroke volume was 115 − 45 = 70 ml. After isovolumic relaxation, left ventricular end diastolic pressure was near atmospheric pressure.

128–130. The answers are: 128-C, 129-D, 130-D. *(Genetics and pathology of chronic myeloprolifera-tive disorder)*
An elevated platelet count and a low white blood cell count are suggestive of chronic myeloproliferative disorder. Malignant lymphoma can be eliminated as a possible diagnosis because of the lack of lymphade-nopathy, and acute leukemia can be eliminated because the lack of blasts on the blood smear. No cough and the normal chest x-ray eliminate pulmonary tuberculosis, which is often associated with myeloproliferative disorders.

Because the cytochemical stains indicate a myeloid disorder, flow cytometric analysis to determine the surface phenotype of peripheral blood and bone marrow cells is not necessary. The leukocyte alkaline phosphatase score is low in chronic myelogenous leukemia (CML) and, therefore, might be useful for differential diagnosis. Since 90% of the patients with CML have a chromosomal translocation resulting in the Philadelphia chromosome, chromosomal evaluation is appropriate. Bone marrow aspiration and biopsy distinguish CML from other chronic myeloproliferative disorders, such as polycythemia vera and agnogenic myeloid metaplasia. Determination of the red blood cell mass distinguishes between polycythemia vera and CML since the red blood cell mass is high in the former but not in the latter.

Approximately 2% to 10% of patients with CML will not have a Philadelphia chromosome but will have a characteristic BCR-*abl* proto-oncogene translocation, which can be detected via nucleic acid hybridization methods. A leukemoid reaction can be excluded because the leukocyte alkaline phophatase levels are not high.

131. The answer is B. *(Chagas disease)*
Patients with chronic Chagas disease present with cardiac conduction defects. The other signs and symptoms listed are classic for several diseases that are endemic in Central and South America, including malaria, visceral and cutaneous leishmaniasis, and amebiasis. Chronic Chagas disease (chronic trypanoso-miasis) results from gradual tissue destruction of the heart, most likely due to damage to myofibrils and the autonomic innervation of the heart. This results in the conduction defects and megacardia, which are hallmarks of the disease. Parasitemia at this point is subpatent; parasites are difficult to detect in either the blood or tissues. Periodic fever and chills are indicative of malaria. Cutaneous and mucocutane-ous lesions are seen in leishmaniasis. Persistent diarrhea and pneumonia can be the result of a number of infectious agents endemic in this region, although these symptoms are not seen in either acute or chronic Chagas disease.

132–139. The answers are: 132-C, 133-E, 134-A, 135-B, 136-D, 137-D, 138-D, 139-C. *(Neuromus-cular transmission and pathophysiology and treatment of myasthenia gravis)*
Edrophonium is a short-acting acetylcholinesterase inhibitor, which increases synaptic acetylcholine (ACh) levels. An increase in muscle strength upon administration of edrophonium is diagnostic of myasthenia gravis.

Myasthenia gravis is a neuromuscular disorder with muscle weakness due to blockade of ACh receptors by autoantibodies to the ACh receptors. The antibody–receptor complex is incapable of responding to ACh and is also rapidly internalized and degraded.

Although the mechanism of action is unclear, aminoglycoside antibiotics and Ca^{2+} have opposing actions in a variety of organ systems. Thus, Ca^{2+} attenuates both the ototoxicity and nephrotoxicity of the aminoglycosides, and the aminoglycosides inhibit presynaptic release of ACh, a process known to be Ca^{2+}-dependent. Intravenous administration of a calcium salt is the preferred treatment for aminoglycoside-induced neuromuscular blockade.

Penicillamine is an effective chelator of heavy metals and is used for the treatment of copper, lead, and mercury poisoning. One of the unusual long-term side effects of penicillamine is a muscle weakness that is indistinguishable from myasthenia gravis.

About 65% of patients with myasthenia gravis have a hyperplastic thymus, and another 10% have a thymic tumor (thymoma). Surgical removal of the thymus and tumors often improves the symptoms dramatically.

Pyridostigmine is the acetylcholinesterase inhibitor most commonly used to treat myasthenia gravis. Isoflurophate (di*iso*propyl phosphorofluoridate; DFP) is an irreversible acetylcholinesterase inhibitor, whose use is limited to ophthalmic applications; pralidoxime is the cholinesterase reactivator that is antidotal for organophosphorus poisoning; and triorthocresylphosphate, the adulterant in Jamaican gin-ger, was the organophosphorus poison responsible for paralysis in thousands of individuals during Prohibition.

Immunosuppression with glucocorticoids is effective in nearly all patients with myasthenia gravis. The therapy presumably works by slowing production of antibodies to the ACh receptors.

140. The answer is E. *(Pharmacokinetics of drugs)*
Nomograms (i.e., body surface area, creatinine clearance) are reliable indicators of appropriate drug dosages in only about 50% of patients with renal insufficiency. Actual peak and trough levels are the only way to guarantee a therapeutic level of antimicrobial agents and avoid toxicity.

141. The answer is C. *(Regulation of peripheral blood flow)*
Compared to other tissue, the lung is relatively unique in having a vasoconstrictor response to hypoxia rather than a vasodilator response. Although the mechanism remains obscure, the rationale seems to be to divert blood flow from poorly ventilated regions of the lung, thus improving the matching of ventilation and perfusion. The vascular bed in the heart, like those in many other organs, dilates to adenosine, and this vasodilator mechanism may be common in its matching of blood flow to local tissue metabolism. The brain has a very well-described and important vasodilator response to carbon dioxide.

142. The answer is C. *(Sterilization; disinfection)*
Bacterial endospores are the life forms most resistant to heat, and they can survive boiling for several minutes. Medically important endospore-formers include members of the genera *Bacillus* and *Clostridium*. Non–spore-formers such as *Escherichia coli* and *Mycobacterium tuberculosis* are more heat-sensitive than spore-formers and are usually killed after several minutes of boiling.

143–144. The answers are: 143-C, 144-C. *(Bacterial meningitis)*
The findings of fever, headache, nuchal rigidity, and lethargy with an acute onset and the lack of dramatic neurologic manifestations suggest acute bacterial meningitis. Viral meningitis causes much of the same symptomatology, but the onset typically is more insidious and the patient usually is less acutely ill. Patients with viral encephalitis display the same general symptomatology as those with viral meningitis, but encephalitis is differentiated by dramatic neurologic manifestations and a much poorer prognosis. Fungal meningitis is more chronic and frequently is seen with other systemic signs of mycotic disease. Brain abscess usually is seen with other foci of infection, and the patient typically has deficits that reflect the location of the lesion.

 Streptococcus pneumoniae is the most common cause of bacterial meningitis among the elderly. *Hemophilus influenzae* type B is the most common cause of bacterial meningitis overall. Its incidence is highest in infants 6 to 12 months old and decreases with age; the incidence of meningitis caused by *H. influenzae* is low in adults. Meningococcal meningitis occurs primarily among young adults, and *Neisseria meningitidis* serogroups A, B, C, and Y cause most cases. *Staphylococcus aureus* occasionally causes meningitis but is a common cause of brain abscess. Raynaud's phenomenon is a peripheral vascular syndrome manifested by sensitivity to cold, livedo reticularis, and acrocyanosis. It occurs primarily in women in their late teens. The etiology is unknown, but the condition is associated with vasospasms.

145–146. The answers are: 145-C, 146-C. *(Neurologic disease topography)*
Guillain-Barré syndrome presents with peripheral sensory defects as well as motor defects, which progress from distal areas of the body to involve more proximal regions. It usually follows a viral illness of unknown origin and affects mostly young people. Loss of deep tendon reflexes is also present. Guillain-Barré syndrome is thought to involve antimyelin autoantibodies against motor neurons that evolve after viral illness or influenza vaccine. There is a progressive mixed motor and sensory loss, even though motor neurons are the target of these antibodies, due to the inflammation of spinal nerves in which both motor and sensory fibers travel together.

 Myasthenia gravis is a disease of the neuromuscular junction and most commonly presents with ocular symptoms, such as ptosis, diplopia, and dysarthria. It manifests as muscle fatigue without sensory symptoms. Deep tendon reflexes are diminished but not lost in this disease. Myasthenia gravis is an autoimmune disease, which involves acetylcholine (ACh) receptors in the postsynaptic neuromuscular junction.

 Poliovirus is a picornavirus, which usually causes an intestinal disease that can progress to viremia and cause the destruction of anterior horn cells of the spinal cord, resulting in paralysis of the innervated muscles. It usually manifests as a purely muscular disorder, and deep tendon reflexes are absent only if the muscles involved in the reflex lose their motor innervation.

147. The answer is D. *(Agnogenic myeloid metaplasia)*
Bone marrow hypocellularity and teardrop-shaped erythrocytes are pathognomonic for agnogenic myeloid metaplasia with myelofibrosis. Leukocyte alkaline phosphatase levels are normal or elevated until the final stages of the disease. The liver does not usually undergo any significant change in size, whereas the spleen is almost always markedly enlarged as it becomes the principal site of extramedullary hematopoiesis.

148. The answer is A. *(Characteristics of warfarin)*
Warfarin affects normal synthesis of clotting factors in the liver, and its anticoagulant effects can be reversed by vitamin K. It is well-absorbed orally but will cross the placenta and may affect the fetus. It is used on a chronic basis for deep venous thrombosis and long-term care postmyocardial infarction because its onset of action is slow. Another useful anticoagulant is heparin, which is a large water-soluble polymer that must be given parenterally and does not cross the placenta. It is primarily used for acute anticoagulant therapy because its onset of action is rapid. It can be reversed by the administration of protamine. The main action of heparin is thought to involve catalyzing the activation of antithrombin III in blood, thereby inhibiting thrombin and factor Xa.

149. The answer is E. *(Antimicrobials and pseudomembranous colitis)*
The patient is likely suffering from antibiotic-associated pseudomembranous colitis (note the patient's diarrhea and deterioration following antibiotic therapy). Sigmoidoscopic examination, Gram stain of feces for white blood cells, a *Clostridium difficile* toxin test, and isolating the patient are appropriate procedures to follow for this patient. However, changing the antibiotic from a cephalosporin to clindamycin is inappropriate because *C. difficile* is not sensitive to clindamycin.

150. The answer is D. *(Cholesterol biosynthesis)*
The rate-limiting and regulated step of cholesterol biosynthesis is the formation of mevalonate from 3-hydroxy-3-methylglutaryl coenzyme A (HMG CoA) catalyzed by HMG CoA reductase. This enzyme is inhibited by dietary cholesterol and endogenously synthesized cholesterol. A vegetarian diet, a diet low in cholesterol, and the administration of a bile acid–sequestering resin all result in a reduced intake of cholesterol, which will not inhibit HMG CoA reductase activity. Familial hypercholesterolemia is a result of a deficiency of low-density lipoprotein (LDL) receptors.

151. The answer is B. *(Fatty acid metabolism; nutrition)*
Because of a methyl group on the third carbon, phytanic acid cannot be metabolized through β-oxidation. Phytanic acid is converted to pristanic acid in peroxisomes by the decarboxylation of the hydroxylated intermediate. Pristanic acid can then be used as a substrate for β-oxidation, as can linoleic acid, arachidonic acid, palmitic acid, and decenoic acid. Phytanic acid is toxic if it is not metabolized.

152. The answer is C. *(Immunology; immunoglobulins)*
Immunoglobulin E (IgE) has a serum half-life of 2 days, making it the shortest lived immunoglobulin. The low serum levels of this class of immunoglobulin are due to both a high affinity for mast cells and basophils and a low rate of synthesis. It is elevated in certain parasitic infections, such as *Ascaris* infections, and is not an agglutinating or complement-fixing antibody.

153. The answer is A. *(Effect of actin and myosin filament overlap on muscle contraction)*
It is generally accepted that maximal contraction of muscle fiber will occur when the overlap between actin filaments and the cross-bridges of the myosin filaments is optimal. At point *D*, the actin filament has pulled all the way out to the end of the myosin filament without overlap, and tension is minimal. As the muscle shortens past the optimal length, *C*, actin filaments tend to overlap each other and the myosin filaments decrease in length *A*, contributing to the decline in contraction at shorter than optimal lengths.

154. The answer is D. *(Serous intermediate ovarian tumor)*
The papillary tumor pictured is a serous intermediate (borderline) tumor of the ovary, which is commonly seen in young women. The tumor behaves in an indolent fashion, with repeated recurrences but rare metastases outside of the abdominal cavity, resulting in a high incidence of intestinal obstruction and long survival. The tumor is characterized by edematous papillae lined by stratified cuboidal to columnar cells, which have atypical cytology. A point of contrast between serous intermediate tumors and serous adenocarcinomas is that intermediate tumors do not invade ovarian stroma.

155–157. The answers are: 155-E, 156-B, 157-E. *(Acute neurologic management; alcohol withdrawal)*
The most important action to take with the ataxic and confused homeless man is to determine what, if any, brain injuries he may have sustained. The scalp wound can be handled initially with a bandage before suturing. If a fracture is suspected, skull films can be obtained after an acute neurologic condition has been ruled out. A serum ethanol level is indicated, and though important, it is not a priority. Hygiene is relevant but not urgent.

Although all of the problems listed in the question must be considered in the differential diagnosis of this patient, the epidural hematoma is the most emergent potential problem listed. An epidural hematoma classically presents as an initial brief period of unconsciousness followed by a lucid period that is followed by unconsciousness. If a sufficient tear of the middle meningeal artery has occurred, death can ensue rapidly. The encephalopathies, including delirium, could progress to coma, but hepatic encephalopathy is not the most urgent choice listed.

Disulfiram (Antabuse) is used as a deterrent to further drinking; it is not a treatment for alcohol withdrawal. Hydration is important to prevent cardiovascular collapse. Benzodiazepines are cross-tolerant with barbiturates and ethanol and permit controlled withdrawal from ethanol. Changes in vital signs, including increased blood pressure, heart rate, and temperature, accompany ethanol withdrawal and should be monitored.

158. The answer is A. (*Myocardial infarction*)
Immediately after a person suffers a myocardial infarction, changes are often evident on an electrocardiogram. Alterations in electrical events in the ventricles, including prolonged depolarization, are common and are manifested by abnormalities in the T wave. Although changes in circulating enzyme levels are helpful for diagnostic and prognostic purposes, they usually occur 6 hours or more after the attack and are more helpful 24 to 72 hours after the myocardial infarction.

159. The answer is D. (*Structure of viruses*)
Viruses have either RNA or DNA, not both. Bacteria in the genus *Chlamydia* contain both types of nucleic acid. Both *Chlamydia* and viruses are obligate intracellular parasites, which depend on the host cell for energy. Since some viruses require arthropod vectors, but other viruses (and *Chlamydia*) do not need arthropod vectors, this is not a dependable differentiating characteristic.

160. The answer is C. (*Genetic code; nucleotides*)
Three nucleotides are required to specify the insertion of an amino acid into a polypeptide chain. These groups of three nucleotides comprise a codon that is represented in the 5' to 3' direction. Because there are four different bases in RNA, the maximum number of codons is sixty-four. Sixty-one of these codons specify the twenty amino acids; some amino acids have more than one. The triplet AUG serves as a start signal, and three triplets that do not code for any amino acid serve as stop signals. The genetic code is virtually universal; all organisms use the same codons to translate their genomes into proteins.

161–162. The answers are: 161-D, 162-A. (*Biostatistical analysis of genetic disorders*)
The patient had a brother with poliodystrophy; therefore, the patient's mother and father must be carriers of the disorder. The patient herself may be heterozygous or homozygous for the dominant allele of the poliodystrophy gene. The probability that a child born to two known carriers will be healthy is 3/4; the probability that such a child is also a carrier is 1/2. Thus,

$$P(\text{patient carrier}|\text{patient healthy}) = \frac{P(\text{patient carrier and patient healthy})}{P(\text{patient healthy})}$$
$$= (1/2) \div (3/4)$$
$$= 2/3$$

In the absence of information on his family history of poliodystrophy, the probability that the patient's husband is a carrier is assumed to equal that of the general population (i.e., 1/20). The probability that both the patient and her husband are carriers is, therefore,

$$P(\text{patient carrier and husband carrier}) = P(\text{patient carrier}) \, P(\text{husband carrier})$$
$$= (2/3) \, (1/20)$$
$$= 1/30$$

163–164. The answers are: 163-B, 164-A. (*Cardiac dynamics*)
The gradient that occurs between the ventricular and aortic systolic pressures is diagnostic of aortic stenosis. The normal aortic valve provides a negligible resistance, and the aortic pressure is nearly identical to the ventricular pressure during the phase of rapid ventricular ejection. A similar picture is seen if right ventricular and pulmonary pressures are measured in the presence of pulmonary valve stenosis, but the pressures are proportionately reduced because of the low resistance of the pulmonary circulation.

Semilunar valve stenosis represents an impediment to the ejection of blood from the ventricle and results in an ejection-type murmur during systole. An ejection murmur is diamond-shaped (i.e., it is a crescendo–decrescendo sound that has maximal intensity in midsystole, when the pressure gradient is largest).

165. The answer is C. *(DNA replication; retroviruses)*
RNA-dependent DNA polymerase synthesizes DNA from an RNA template and is essential for the replication of retroviruses, not cells, and is, therefore, not a potential target of the new drug. Topoisomerase II relaxes supercoiled DNA. RNA polymerase synthesizes a primer fragment for DNA-dependent DNA polymerase. DNA ligase anneals the Okazaki fragments on the lagging strand of DNA synthesis.

166. The answer is B. *(Mitochondrial intracellular localization)*
Mitochondria typically exist in cell areas that use substantial amounts of adenosine triphosphate (ATP). They are abundant in the apices of ciliated cells because the beating action of cilia consumes ATP. They also exist in apices of cells that have a microvillous brush border such as the cells lining the proximal thick segment of the kidneys, because solute transport and pinocytosis of proteins in the glomerular filtrate consume energy and, therefore, require ATP. Mitochondria are distributed evenly throughout the cytoplasm of smooth muscle cells, steroid-secreting cells, skeletal muscle cells, and liver parenchymal cells rather than existing in apical concentrations.

167. The answer is C. *(Neuromuscular transmission)*
Motoneurons innervate many skeletal muscle fibers. In large muscles, thousands of fibers may be innervated by one neuron. However, each fiber receives only one axon terminal. Depolarization of the nerve terminal releases acetylcholine (ACh) into the synaptic cleft, where it binds directly to Na^+ channels, causing an end-plate potential. The end-plate itself is not electrically excitable, but passive spreading of end-plate potential to a nearby membrane leads to propagation of the action potential and contraction of all muscle fibers innervated by the motoneuron. When ACh is the neurotransmitter, termination of transmission is accomplished by hydrolysis via acetylcholinesterase.

168. The answer is C. *(Herpes simplex virus infection of the nervous system)*
"Cold sores" are caused by the herpes simplex virus (HSV), which usually infects the lips, philtrum, and the areas around the nares of affected individuals. After the primary infection, HSV establishes a latent state in the ganglia of cranial nerve (CN) V where the second (CN V_2) and third (CN V_3) branches of this nerve innervate the areas described above. CN VII is not infected by this virus.

169. The answer is B. *(Characteristics of chronic type B gastritis)*
Chronic type B gastritis is four times more common than type A (fundal) gastritis, the form of chronic gastritis in which there are circulating antibodies to the parietal cells and intrinsic factor. Type B gastritis may result from chronic alcohol or aspirin use, bile reflux, ulcer disease, or postgastrectomy states. Type A is found in elderly individuals and individuals with pernicious anemia. Levels of gastrin tend to be low, and there may be antibodies to gastrin-producing cells in type B gastritis, in contrast to type A gastritis. In type B gastritis, the stomach wall loses its rugal folds and becomes flattened, glazed, and red.

170. The answer is E. *(DNA replication)*
DNA replication begins at specific sites. In *Escherichia coli,* DNA replication starts at a unique origin and proceeds sequentially in opposite directions. Because of the size of the eukaryotic genome, multiple replication origins are important for timely DNA replication. DNA polymerase cannot start chains de novo; all known DNA polymerases add mononucleotides to the 3' hydroxyl end of an RNA primer, or, as in the case of adenovirus replication, DNA synthesis begins from a serine residue on a protein primet. DNA replication occurs during the S phase of the cell cycle.

171. The answer is C. *(Diagnosis of syphilis)*
A Venereal Disease Research Laboratory (VDRL) test and darkfield examination would be the most appropriate combination of tests for determining the cause of the penile lesion. A painless penile lesion that is crateriform, moist, and indurated is suggestive of primary syphilis. The organism responsible, *Treponema pallidum,* cannot be cultured or detected by Gram stain. It can, however, be visualized by darkfield observation of scrapings from the lesion. Some, but not all, patients with primary syphilis have serologic evidence of infection, readily detected by the VDRL test. The fluorescent treponemal antibody absorption (FTA-ABS) test is only used to confirm diagnosis and is not appropriate here.

172. The answer is B. *(Radiolabeled uptake)*
One of the best methods for measuring cellular proliferation is measuring the uptake of radiolabeled nucleic acid. Dividing cells require nucleotides for DNA synthesis, and the uptake of labeled thymidine and its incorporation in DNA is an excellent indicator of cell proliferation. Uracil, which is only used in RNA synthesis, except for some reconstituted through a salvage pathway, would not be indicative of cell division, only of messenger RNA (mRNA) synthesis. Likewise, uptake and incorporation of radiolabeled

methionine would involve protein synthesis, not cell division. Trypan blue exclusion is used for quantitating viability and would not be useful in this experiment.

173. The answer is B. *(Neuroanatomy)*
The limbic system is concerned with unconscious biologic drives and emotions and, hence, is considered the most primitive part of the brain. It contains the limbic lobe, hippocampus, anterior thalamic nucleus, hypothalamus, and the amygdala.

174. The answer is E. *(RNA structure and function)*
In eukaryotes, messenger RNA (mRNA) is formed in the nucleus and must be exported into the cytosol for translation. The initial product of transcription includes all of the introns and flanking regions, which must be removed by splicing before correct translation can occur. The splicing reaction involves hydrolysis of phosphodiester bonds and formation of new phosphodiester bonds within the mRNA molecule. Other processing reactions include additions at both the 5′ and 3′ ends. A guanosine triphosphate (GTP) molecule is added in reverse orientation to form a cap at the 5′ end, and the cap is further modified by the addition of methyl groups. A polyadenylate tail is added at the 3′ end.

175–176. The answers are: 175-C, 176-C. *(Eukaryotic and viral commonalities)*
Arenaviruses are multisegmented RNA viruses with inclusion granules in the virions that contain ribosomes derived from their host cells. Although arenaviruses have envelopes, this is a trait shared by many viruses, including herpesviruses and orthomyxoviruses. Likewise, many viruses have multiple genomic segments, including orthomyxoviruses and paramyxoviruses. Only arenaviruses contain ribosomes; in fact, the Latin word "arena" means sand. The presence of ribosome-containing granules makes the virus look grainy under the electron microscope.

To determine if the unknown virus is an arenavirus, it is important to locate the characteristic ribosomes. To test for the presence of ribosomes in virions, it would be necessary to supply ribosomal substrates to virion fractions and test the ability of these fractions to translate cellular messenger RNA (mRNA) and radiolabeled amino acids into proteins that could be isolated on a detergent (SDS) gel. Gel electrophoresis and ethidium bromide are useful for separating and staining double-stranded DNA fragments, since ethidium bromide is an intercalating dye for DNA. Light microscopy with a hematoxylin–eosin stain would be useful for viewing viruses with known inclusion-body forming properties but not useful in determining if an unknown virus is an arenavirus.

177–178. The answers are: 177-B, 178-B. *(Lyme disease)*
Lyme disease is a recently described tick-borne disease in which the infectious agent is a spirochete, *Borrelia burgdorferi*. Erythema chronicum migrans and positive antibody to the spirochete are presumed to be diagnostic for this condition, which may be manifested by flu-like symptoms that may ultimately progress towards arthritic, cardiac, and central nervous system (CNS) symptoms. The causative spirochete is sensitive to several antibiotics, including penicillin, tetracycline, and erythromycin.

179. The answer is B. *(Histopathology of meningiomas)*
The tumor in the photomicrograph is a meningioma, which has a marked predilection for women and arises from the pia–arachnoid cells of the leptomeninges. It is usually well circumscribed and may have a hyperostotic reaction of overlying bone associated with it. The tumor cells are arranged in whorls or nests, and they are frequently observed with concentric calcified concretions called psammoma bodies, as can be seen on the *right* of the photomicrograph.

180. The answer is A. *(Pathophysiology of anemia)*
The result of a diet deficient in vitamin B_{12} or folate can be macrocytic, normochromic anemia with characteristic hypersegmented neutrophils. Anemia due to folate or vitamin B_{12} deficiency often also presents with thrombocytopenia and agranulocytopenia. Microcytic, hypochromic erythrocytes are observed in iron deficiency anemia and thalassemia minor. Additionally, basophilic stippling and target cells can be seen in thalassemia minor. In sickle cell crisis, the anemia is normocytic and normochromic, as is the anemia associated with hemorrhage.

181. The answer is C. *(Microscopic features of hemangioma)*
The hepatic neoplasm pictured is a benign cavernous hemangioma. This is the most common mesenchymal tumor of the liver, and, if it reaches an enormous size, it may be associated with a bruit over the liver and thrombocytopenia due to venous stasis and in situ thrombosis. The neoplasm is comprised of dilated vascular spaces lined by flattened, cytologically bland endothelial cells *(at right)*. Angiosarcomas of the liver have highly aggressive behavior and usually have foci of hemorrhage and necrosis. They are

associated with particular carcinogens, one of which is Thorotrast, a radioactive medium widely used 50 years ago.

182. The answer is C. *(Thalamic connections)*
The pulvinar nucleus receives input from the superior colliculus and pretectal areas and projects to visual cortex areas 18 and 19. It does not connect with the basal ganglia.

183. The answer is A. *(Structure and function of amino acids in proteins)*
The physical and chemical properties of the peptide reflect the properties of the constituent amino acids. At pH 7.4, the positive and negative charges of the α-amino and α-carboxyl terminal groups cancel one another. The side chains of the two aspartate and one glutamate residues are negatively charged; the side chain of arginine is positively charged. Cysteine and methionine both contain sulfur atoms. Any of the amino acids containing a hydrogen atom attached to a sulfur, nitrogen, or oxygen atom, or containing an atom with an unshared pair of electrons, could form hydrogen bonds. The amino acids valine, phenylalanine, methionine, and cysteine contribute hydrophobic character to the peptide. The specificity of chymotrypsin is for peptide bonds in which the carboxyl group is donated by an aromatic amino acid.

184. The answer is C. *(Pharmacologic treatment of arrhythmias)*
Lidocaine is often the drug of first choice for the treatment of ventricular arrhythmia. It suppresses Na^+ currents in the infarct area that have abnormal resting membrane potentials and elevated K^+ levels. If lidocaine fails, the most frequently chosen agent is another Na^+-channel blocker, procainamide. The Ca^{2+}-channel blockers (diltiazem, verapamil) and β-blockers (propranolol) have a greater effect on supraventricular disturbances in which slow Ca^{2+} channels are involved more significantly than Na^+ channels.

185. The answer is D. *(Renal cell carcinoma)*
The renal mass pictured is classic clear cell carcinoma of the kidney. The cells have round to oval nuclei and inconspicuous nucleoli. The cytoplasm is abundant; it is clear due to the large amounts of glycogen and lipid within these cells (the glycogen accounts for the yellow color). Renal cell carcinomas may be hemorrhagic, and they tend to invade the renal veins and inferior vena cava, from which they may metastasize to the bones and lungs.

186. The answer is B. *(Urea cycle)*
The nitrogens in urea, the disposal form of ammonia, come from ammonia and aspartate. Ammonia reacts with carbon dioxide and adenosine triphosphate (ATP) to form carbamoyl phosphate in a reaction catalyzed by carbamoyl phosphate synthetase (ammonia). This enzyme requires N-acetylglutamate as a positive allosteric effector. Without this reaction, urea would not be formed, and ammonia levels would be high. The next step in the urea cycle is the reaction of carbamoyl phosphate with ornithine to form citrulline. In the absence of carbamoyl phosphate, ornithine levels are high, citrulline is undetectable, and neither argininosuccinate nor arginine is formed.

187. The answer is B. *(Neurologic assessment)*
Cerebellar disease manifests as dystonia to palpation but does not alter grip strength. Pain elicited by touching the chin to the chest is known as Brudzinski's sign and usually indicates inflammation of the meninges. Cerebellar disease is indicated by decreased resistance of the limbs to passive movement. Deep tendon reflexes continue for longer than usual, and in the patellar tendon, this is known as the "pendular knee jerk" due to the motion of the limb when the reflex is elicited. Patients with cerebellar disease also show voluntary ataxia, dysdiadochokinesia, nystagmus, and dysarthria of the larynx. Cerebellar lesions usually affect the ipsilateral body.

188–191. The answers are: 188-A, 189-C, 190-B, 191-A. *(Pelvic innervation)*
Afferent nerves from the pelvic viscera travel along autonomic pathways. Afferents from the ovary, testis, upper to middle ureter, uterine tubes, urinary bladder, and uterine body travel along the least splanchnic nerve to the lower thoracic segment and along the lumbar splanchnic nerves to the upper lumbar segments of the spinal cord; thus, pain is referred to the inguinal and pubic regions as well as the lateral and anterior aspects of the thigh. Afferents from the epididymis, uterine cervix, and distal ureter travel along the pelvic splanchnic nerves to the midsacral spinal segments; thus, pain is referred to the perineum, posterior thigh, and leg.

192–196. The answers are: 192-C, 193-A, 194-E, 195-B, 196-D. *(Placental anatomy)*
The placenta consists of a decidual plate (*C*) facing the endometrium and a chorionic plate (*E*) facing the fetus. The decidual plate and chorionic plate are fused at the margins of the discoid placenta. These two plates are interconnected by cytotrophoblastic cell columns (*B*). Large numbers of chorionic villi (*D*) project away from them into the intervillous space (*A*). Maternal blood vessels end on the decidual plate and pour maternal blood into the intervillous space. Maternal blood directly bathes the chorionic villi. Thus, the human placenta is said to be a hemochorial placenta.

197–201. The answers are: 197-A, 198-D, 199-E, 200-C, 201-B. *(Cranial vasculature)*
The foramen spinosum transmits the middle meningeal artery (*A*), a branch of the maxillary artery. The carotid canal (*D*) transmits the internal carotid artery, while the jugular foramen (*E*) contains the internal jugular vein in addition to the glossopharyngeal, vagus, and spinal accessory nerves. Each posterior condylar canal (*C*) transmits a large emissary vein. The vertebral arteries enter the cranial cavity through the foramen magnum (*B*) along with the spinal accessory nerve; the spinal cord also transmits the foramen magnum.

202–206. The answers are: 202-C, 203-E, 204-B, 205-E, 206-A. *(Regulation of thyroid hormone synthesis)*
Regulation of thyroid hormone synthesis is a complex pathway. The anterior pituitary secretion of thyroid-stimulating hormone (TSH, or thyrotropin) is controlled by the hypothalamic hormone, thyrotropin-releasing hormone (TRH). TRH is a tripeptide whose synthesis may be stimulated by such conditions as stress, trauma, or cold temperatures. TSH affects all aspects of thyroid gland physiology, including stimulation of thyroxine (T_4) secretion and to a lesser extent triiodothyronine (T_3) secretion in the presence of sufficient iodine. T_4 is activated to T_3 by peripheral deiodination. In certain forms of hyperthyroidism, high circulating levels of thyroid hormone suppress the synthesis of TSH via a direct negative feedback pathway. Propylthiouracil and other antithyroid agents are useful adjuvants to surgical or radiologic removal of the hypersecreting thyroid gland in such conditions as Graves' disease. These agents prevent thyroperoxidase oxidation in the thyroid gland and, perhaps, peripheral deiodination of T_4, resulting in a decreased circulating level and activity of T_4. Levothyroxine is a synthetic, pure compound that is used for the therapy of myxedema, cretinism, and other forms of hypothyroidism. It is available for oral use.

207–210. The answers are: 207-B, 208-D, 209-E, 210-C. *(Sleep architecture)*
In narcolepsy, sleep attacks are sleep-onset rapid eye movement (REM) periods that intrude into wakefulness. The motor paralysis component of sleep-onset REM periods that are associated with narcolepsy is called cataplexy. REM sleep normally occurs about 90 minutes after sleep onset, but in major depression, it occurs after only 45 minutes. There are also increased amounts of REM throughout the night in depressed individuals. Vaginal lubrication and penile tumescence occur spontaneously during normal REM sleep. Night terrors are characterized by partial awakening in terror from stages III and IV (when delta waves occur) of slow-wave sleep (SWS).

211–216. The answers are: 211-A, 212-C, 213-B, 214-F, 215-E, 216-D. *(Gross and microscopic appearances of neoplasms)*
Grossly, the squamous cell carcinoma is a firm, white–tan mass, approximately 2 cm in diameter. Histologically, the neoplasm displays nuclei having hyperchromatic coarse chromatin; nucleoli may or may not be observed. The tumor may be indolent, with a prominent host response consisting of inflammation and fibroblastic proliferation.

Grossly, the bronchioalveolar adenocarcinoma is white and granular and ranges from several millimeters to several centimeters in diameter. On chest x-ray, the lesion may resemble "fluffy" infiltrates of pneumonia. This tumor also follows a rather indolent course, but the multicentric foci, which appear to result from aerogenic spread, limit resectability.

Grossly, the type of adenocarcinoma usually seen often appears as a tan mass between 1 cm and 3 cm in diameter. Histologically, the tumor cell cytoplasm is pale-staining and may contain mucin vacuoles. The nuclei are round or oval, with delicate chromatin patterns and prominent nucleoli. This tumor often metastasizes early to the brain.

Grossly, carcinoid often appears as a fleshy, brown, intrabronchial polyp. Histologically, the tumor grows in a pattern of clusters or ribbons of cells. The neurosecretory granules may contain neuron-specific enolase, bombesin, serotonin, calcitonin, gastrin, adrenocorticotropic hormone (ACTH), and somatostatin, among other materials. A carcinoid often arises in the appendix and terminal ileum.

The rapidly replicating small, primitive-appearing cells of small cell (oat cell) carcinoma have finely stippled nuclei, a high nuclear:cytoplasm ratio, and nucleoli that are not prominent. The small, dense neurosecretory granules may contain markers such as neuron-specific enolase, bombesin, calcitonin, somatostatin, vasoactive intestinal polypeptide (VIP), or ACTH. Long-term survival is poor due to extensive metastases to the liver, brain, bone, or adrenal glands by the time of diagnosis.

The large cell carcinoma is usually 3 cm to 6 cm in diameter. It is a white–tan tumor that is partially necrotic or cavitating. In addition to the leukemoid reaction, the presence of this tumor may also be manifested by elevated serum levels of the β-chain of chorionic gonadotropin.

217–221. The answers are: 217-B, 218-A, 219-E, 220-C, 221-D. _(Cell organelle structure and function)_
The Golgi complex (_B_) is composed of flattened membranous sacs and functions in protein glycosylation, membrane recycling, and sorting and targeting of proteins. Introns are regions of DNA that are transcribed but not translated. In the nucleus (_A_), introns are cleaved from primary RNA transcripts to produce mature messenger RNA (mRNA). Ribosomes are composed of ribosomal RNA (rRNA), which is synthesized in the nucleolus (_E_) of the cell by RNA polymerase I. Smooth endoplasmic reticulum (_C_) has various functions, including steroid synthesis; calcium homeostasis; and lipid, cholesterol, and drug metabolism. Adenosine triphosphate (ATP) is synthesized by glycolysis in the cytosol and by oxidative phosphorylation in the mitochondria (_D_).

222–226. The answers are: 222-B, 223-D, 224-E, 225-A, 226-C. _(Transport proteins)_
The functions of transport proteins can be divided into three general classes: the control of diffusion into the tissues; the highly specific recognition of molecules; and the removal of toxins. Transferrin helps in transporting iron to storage and utilization sites in the bone marrow. The damage that free iron can cause to tissues other than the marrow is prevented when it is bound by transferrin. Transcobalamin binds vitamin B_{12} and prevents it from degrading while it is being transported to storage and utilization sites in tissues with high cellular turnover rates. Albumin is the main plasma protein responsible for the maintenance of plasma osmotic pressure. Haptoglobin is a plasma protein that binds free hemoglobin in the blood and delivers it to the liver for recycling. The degree of intravascular hemolysis is determined by measuring the levels of depleted free forms of haptoglobin in the blood.

227–231. The answers are: 227-A, 228-B, 229-B, 230-A, 231-A. _(Vitamin deficiency)_
Pellagra, a disease affecting the skin (dermatitis), the gastrointestinal tract (diarrhea), and the central nervous system (CNS) [dementia], is the result of a niacin deficiency. Because niacin can be formed from tryptophan, an essential amino acid, dietary treatment of pellagra must take into consideration daily allowances for both niacin and tryptophan. Endemic pellagra is no longer a common occurrence; however, it is a manifestation of two disorders of tryptophan metabolism, Hartnup disease and the carcinoid syndrome. Hartnup disease is an autosomal recessive defect in which patients have a reduced ability to convert tryptophan to niacin. In the carcinoid syndrome, dietary tryptophan is metabolized in the hydroxylation pathway (a minor pathway), leaving little tryptophan for the formation of niacin. Administration of large amounts of niacin can cure the pellagra associated with these conditions.

Beriberi is a severe thiamine deficiency syndrome associated with malnutrition endemic to areas where there is a high intake of highly milled (polished) rice. Clinical characteristics of this deficiency range from cardiovascular and neurologic lesions to emotional disturbances. Cardiovascular changes include right-sided enlargement (dilatation), tachycardia, and "high-output" cardiac failure. Neuromuscular manifestations include peripheral neuropathy (neuritis), weakness, fatigue, and an impaired capacity to do work. Edema and anorexia are also characteristic. In the United States, thiamine deficiency is seen primarily in association with chronic alcoholism, which leads to Wernicke's encephalopathy, which presents with the classic triad of confusion, ataxia, and ophthalmoplegia. In thiamine deficiency, motor and sensory peripheral nerve lesions are marked by neuromuscular findings of numbness and tingling of the legs and atrophy and weakness of the muscles of the extremities compounded by the loss of reflexes. Mental depression may also accompany these findings. The dementia caused by niacin deficiency results from degeneration of the ganglion cells of the brain, accompanied by degeneration of the fibers of the spinal cord.

232–236. The answers are: 232-E, 233-A, 234-B, 235-D, 236-C. _(Endocrine syndromes)_
Bartter's syndrome is a form of secondary hyperaldosteronism in which excessive renin production occurs. The hyperreninemia results from hyperplasia of renal juxtaglomerular cells, which secrete renin primarily in response to decreased arterial blood pressure in afferent arterioles and increased renal sympathetic nerve activity.

Sheehan's syndrome, or postpartum pituitary necrosis, results from the infarction of the anterior lobe of the pituitary gland. Sheehan's syndrome usually is precipitated by obstetric hemorrhage or shock; however, it also can occur in nonpregnant women as well as in men. The infarct usually causes the destruction of 95% to 99% of the anterior lobe.

Cushing's syndrome is characterized by a prolonged overproduction of cortisol. The pituitary gland regulates the synthesis of adrenal cortisol by secreting adrenocorticotropic hormone (ACTH). The secretion of ACTH is regulated by corticotropin-releasing hormone (CRH), which is produced in the hypothalamus. Possible causes of Cushing's syndrome include: ACTH-producing pituitary neoplasm; CRH-producing hypothalamic neoplasm; adrenal cortisol-producing neoplasm; and ectopic ACTH- or CRH-producing neoplasm. Cushing's syndrome can be caused iatrogenically by long-term glucocorticoid therapy.

Waterhouse-Friderichsen syndrome is most often caused by meningococcemia and is characterized by extensive cutaneous petechiae, purpura, and hemorrhages. Skin lesions appear shortly after the onset of an infectious febrile reaction, and the patient may go into circulatory collapse and die within 24 hours. In addition to lesions, extensive internal hemorrhages are present, particularly in the adrenal glands.

Conn's syndrome, or primary hyperaldosteronism, is associated with hypernatremia, hypokalemia, alkalosis, potassium wasting, and low levels of renin.

237–240. The answers are: 237-A, 238-B, 239-B, 240-D. *(Small intestine)*
Differences between segments of the small intestine are subtle; however, several distinguishing features aid identification. The jejunum contains well-developed plicae circulares, tall arteriae rectae, and few arterial arcades. The ileum has rudimentary plicae circulares, short arteriae rectae, and many arterial arcades. Meckel's diverticulum, a remnant of the embryonic vitelline duct, is present in the ileum in approximately 3% of the population. Appendices epiploicae (fat-filled tags) are diagnostic for the large bowel only.

241–244. The answers are: 241-C, 242-A, 243-D, 244-E. *(Neurophysiology and visual science)*
Presbyopia (impairment of vision due to old age) is caused by a decrease in the elasticity of the lens. As a result, the eyes are unable to accommodate for near vision. Another condition associated with aging is cataracts, in which the lens becomes progressively less transparent. Myopia is caused by an overall refractive power that is too great for the axial length of the eyeball. It causes distant objects to be focused in front of the retina and can be corrected by a diverging lens. In hyperopia, the overall refractive power is too low for the axial length of the eyeball, and so the eyes must continuously accommodate to see distant objects clearly.

245–248. The answers are: 245-B, 246-E, 247-A, 248-C. *(Quantitative dose–response curves)*
The figure on the *left* represents an ideal concentration–response curve for a drug and shows the typical hyperbolic effect. The concentration that gives the half-maximal effect (K_D) can be estimated from the figure, but the maximal effect cannot easily be determined because of the hyperbolic nature of the data. The figure on the *right* is a mathematical transformation of these data to a linear form that is more useful—a Scatchard plot that allows the maximal effect to be determined from the intercept at the X axis. The concentration of K_D is the reciprocal of the slope.

249–253. The answers are: 249-C, 250-A, 251-B, 252-E, 253-D. *(Cell division)*
The beginning of prophase is marked by the appearance of chromosomes within the nucleus. Throughout prophase, the chromosomes condense further; dissolution of the nuclear envelope marks the end of this phase. During metaphase, the kinetochore becomes attached to tubulin, the major component of the mitotic spindle. Metaphase is marked by the alignment of chromosomes along the equatorial (metaphase) plane. The next stage of cell division is anaphase, and it is marked by the separation of the centromeres. By the addition of tubulin to the mitotic spindle, the chromosomes are drawn toward opposite poles of the cell. Anaphase ends when the chromosomes are clustered at opposite poles of the cell. During the final stage, telophase, the chromosomes uncoil, the nuclear envelope reforms, and the cell divides. As the cell divides, the cytoplasm also divides by a process known as cytokinesis; these processes continue until two daughter cells are produced. During telophase, cell division is thought to occur by the constriction of a ring of actin filaments.

254–258. The answers are: 254-A, 255-D, 256-C, 257-B, 258-E. *(Systemic blood pressure)*
Normal blood pressure is 140/90 or less in adults. If only the systolic pressure is elevated, this is called isolated systolic hypertension; if the word "hypertension" is used without further qualification, it is presumed that both the systolic and the diastolic elements are high. The normal response to standing upright is a slight rise in pulse rate, a small drop in systolic pressure, and a small rise in diastolic pressure.

With volume depletion, both the systolic and the diastolic pressure often drop more considerably; however, if the host has intact vascular reflexes, the pressures may be maintained, or nearly so, by a marked increase in heart rate. This is the situation depicted in the 59-year-old man, where the pressures are almost steady, but at the cost of a 23-beat rise in heart rate. If the pressures drop and there is no compensatory increase in heart rate, the autonomic response is dysfunctional, as shown in the 68-year-old man.

Practice Examination II

QUESTIONS

Directions: Each of the numbered items or incomplete statements in this section is followed by answers or by completions of the statement. Select the **one** lettered answer or completion that is **best** in each case.

1. Of the following types of proteins, all exhibit a protein structure common for physiologic receptors or components of cellular signal transduction system EXCEPT

(A) ion channels
(B) protein kinases
(C) guanylate cyclases
(D) guanosine triphosphate (GTP)–binding proteins (G proteins)
(E) metallothionin

2. All of the following statements about γ-aminobutyric acid (GABA) are true EXCEPT

(A) its receptor is coupled to a benzodiazepine receptor
(B) it is a widely distributed inhibitory neurotransmitter
(C) its activity is increased in hepatic encephalopathy
(D) its activity is increased with antispasticity drugs
(E) its activity is decreased with antiseizure drugs

Questions 3–7

A child presents to the pediatrician for evaluation of "difficulty walking." Examination reveals a waddling gait, proximal muscle weakness, pseudohypertrophy of the calf muscles, and a Gower maneuver upon standing from a sitting position. A tentative diagnosis of Duchenne muscular dystrophy (DMD) is made, pending the results of serum enzyme studies, electromyography, and muscle biopsy. A family pedigree is illustrated below.

3. According to the pedigree, the mode of inheritance of DMD is

(A) autosomal recessive
(B) autosomal dominant
(C) X-linked
(D) nonpenetrant
(E) none of the above

4. What is the chance that the mother is a carrier for DMD?

(A) 25%
(B) 50%
(C) 75%
(D) 100%
(E) None of the above

5. What is the chance that the next male child will carry the gene that causes the disease?

(A) None
(B) 50%
(C) 75%
(D) 100%
(E) None of the above

6. The defect in DMD involves a mutation in the gene coding for which of the following proteins?

(A) Actin
(B) Dystrophin
(C) Spectrin
(D) Tropomyosin
(E) None of the above

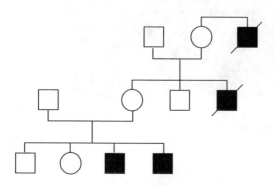

7. Some DMD can be diagnosed prenatally by which of the following techniques?

(A) Genetic probes

(B) Linkage analysis

(C) Western blot

(D) Southern blot

(E) None of the above

8. All of the following nephritides are associated with hypocomplementemia EXCEPT

(A) immunoglobulin A (IgA) nephropathy

(B) mesangioproliferative glomerulonephropathy

(C) serum sickness

(D) systemic lupus erythematosus (SLE)

(E) vasculitis

9. The violaceous skin nodule apparent in the photomicrograph below, which was taken from a young individual, is most likely

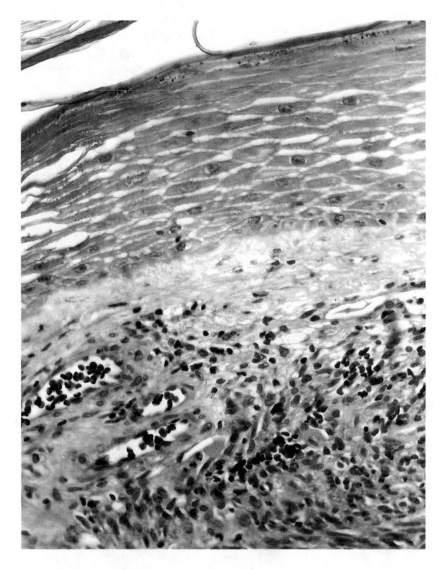

(A) seen on the back of infants' necks

(B) a highly malignant pigmented melanoma

(C) seen in homosexual men

(D) due to radiation therapy that was administered over 10 years ago

10. Which one of the following statements concerning referred pain is true?

(A) Pain from the transverse colon is usually referred to a midline area below the umbilicus

(B) Somatic pain is usually referred in a diffuse, poorly localized pattern

(C) Diaphragmatic pain is usually referred to the inguinal area

(D) The mechanism of referred pain is well understood

Questions 11–13

An 18-year-old college freshman has been "acting strangely" for several months, according to his roommates. His grades are deteriorating, and he avoids social interactions. He talks about being the devil's accomplice. He is unshaven, and his clothes are messy.

11. The first diagnosis to consider with this patient is

(A) schizophrenia

(B) mania

(C) schizoaffective disorder

(D) major depression

(E) phencyclidine psychosis

12. Further history reveals periods of staring spells and olfactory hallucinations. Based on these symptoms, the physician should order which of the following tests?

(A) Bender Gestalt test

(B) Thematic Apperception test

(C) Electroencephalogram

(D) Halstead-Reitan battery

(E) Brain stem evoked potentials

13. A reasonable medication trial for complex partial seizures is

(A) haloperidol

(B) carbamazepine

(C) imipramine

(D) alprazolam

(E) clonidine

14. The term that describes the adherence of neutrophils and monocytes to the vascular endothelium prior to movement into the extravascular space is

(A) margination

(B) diapedesis

(C) pavementing

(D) emigration

(E) clotting

15. A fluorescent probe that binds to glucocorticoid receptors is applied to cells. The probe is freely diffusible throughout the cell and has no effect on the glucocorticoid receptor. If the cell has not been previously stimulated by glucocorticoids, where is the most intense fluorescence?

(A) Cell membrane

(B) Cytosol

(C) Nuclear membrane

(D) Nucleus

(E) Nucleus and cytosol

16. All of the following human leukocyte antigen (HLA) associations are matched correctly EXCEPT

(A) rheumatoid arthritis—HLA-DR4

(B) primary Sjögrens syndrome—HLA-DR3

(C) postgonococcal arthritis—HLA-B27

(D) 21-hydroxylase deficiency—HLA-DR4

(E) chronic active hepatitis—HLA-DR3

17. A middle-aged woman presented with a throbbing headache and bilateral tenderness over her forehead. Knobby cords were palpated at the sides and were biopsied. The tissue is pictured in the micrograph below. The correct diagnosis is

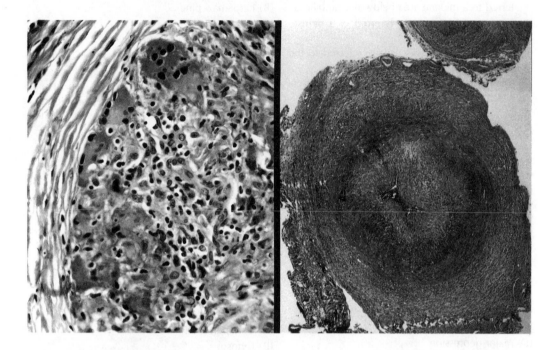

(A) temporal arteritis

(B) foreign body giant cell reaction to an injected substance

(C) Mönckeberg's arteriosclerosis

(D) Takayasu's arteritis

18. Cromolyn sodium is now the first-line agent for the treatment of mild to moderate asthma, especially asthma in children associated with allergenic causes. Although its mechanism of action is unclear, cromolyn sodium's widespread use is due to its

(A) bioavailability after oral administration

(B) direct bronchodilating effect, making it useful in acute emergencies

(C) prophylactic potential secondary to inhibition of the release of inflammatory mediators

(D) immediate effect to reduce bronchospasm

(E) antimuscarinic effects

Questions 19–20

A 50-year-old woman complains of increasing fatigue over the past 2 weeks. She has a history of ovarian carcinoma and has received treatment with several courses of cyclophosphamide during the past 3 years, with her last course of treatment given 1 month ago. Physical examination shows slight hepatic enlargement. One examiner thinks the patient has some excess abdominal fluid. Laboratory examination reveals a white blood count of 2000 cells/μl, with 10% polymorphonuclear leukocytes and 90% lymphocytes. The hemoglobin concentration is 9 g/dl, and the platelet count is 50,000/μl.

19. The differential diagnosis of the cause of this patient's pancytopenia includes all of the following EXCEPT

(A) chronic lymphocytic leukemia

(B) acute myelogenous leukemia

(C) recurrent ovarian carcinoma

(D) cyclophosphamide toxicity

(E) aplastic anemia

20. Further evaluation of this patient requires all of the following studies EXCEPT

(A) radiographic studies of the abdomen

(B) cytologic examination of ascites

(C) bone marrow aspiration and biopsy

(D) immunoglobulin gene rearrangement studies

(E) liver function studies

21. Asthma is characterized by an increased responsiveness of the trachea and bronchi to various stimuli and is manifested by widespread narrowing of the airway. Results of pulmonary function tests during an acute asthma attack will demonstrate all of the following EXCEPT

(A) decreased forced expiratory volume in 1 second (FEV_1)

(B) increased forced vital capacity (FVC)

(C) decreased FEV_1/FVC

(D) normal or increased total lung capacity (TLC)

22. A 62-year-old man experiences crushing substernal chest pain. After 4 days of circulatory support in the intensive care unit, he dies. Histologic study of his heart would show all of the following findings EXCEPT

(A) coagulative necrosis

(B) liquefactive necrosis

(C) hypereosinophilic wavy fibers

(D) neutrophilic infiltrate

Questions 23–26

A patient presents with epigastric and right upper quadrant pain. The pain is most intense 2–4 hours after eating and is reduced by the ingestion of antacids. The patient states that he has passed black tarry stools (melena) within the last week.

23. In considering gastric ulcer in the differential diagnosis, the physician should note all of the following risk factors EXCEPT

(A) smoking

(B) elevated secretion of hydrochloric acid (HCl)

(C) caffeine

(D) heredity

(E) gender

24. Fiberoptic endoscopy reveals a yellowish crater surrounded by a rim of erythema that is 3 cm distal to the pylorus. Accordingly, an ulcer has been identified in the patient's

(A) fundus

(B) antrum

(C) duodenum

(D) jejunum

(E) ileum

25. Hypertrophy of which of the following submucosal structures often accompanies denudation of the epithelium in peptic ulcer?

(A) Brunner's glands

(B) Meissner's plexus

(C) Auerbach's plexus

(D) Peyer's patches

(E) Paneth's cells

26. Possible pharmacotherapy for this patient may include

(A) bethanechol

(B) diphenhydramine

(C) indomethacin

(D) ranitidine

(E) dexamethasone

27. The most important prognostic factor for human cancer is

(A) the patient's age
(B) tumor stage
(C) lymphocytic infiltration
(D) vascular invasion
(E) the mitotic index

28. The following elements of the adult brain develop from the telencephalon EXCEPT the

(A) corpus striatum
(B) internal capsule
(C) occipital lobe
(D) hippocampus
(E) thalamus

29. Growth hormone (GH; somatotropic hormone; somatotropin) is synthesized and stored in large amounts in the anterior pituitary gland (adenohypophysis). Which of the following statements accurately describes GH?

(A) It is secreted continuously
(B) Synthesis is stimulated by the action of somatostatin
(C) Receptors have a limited distribution outside the central nervous system (CNS)
(D) It stimulates cartilage and bone growth via somatomedin
(E) It has a proinsulin-like effect in addition to its other actions

30. Each statement below concerning the contraction of myofibrils in skeletal muscle is true EXCEPT

(A) the size of the A band decreases
(B) the size of the H band decreases
(C) the size of the I band decreases
(D) thin filaments penetrate the A band
(E) Z disks are drawn closer to the A band

31. A 29-year-old intravenous drug abuser presented with bilateral fluffy lung infiltrates. A transbronchial biopsy was performed. A Grocott-Gomori methenamine-silver nitrate stain was performed on the lung tissue (pictured below). The diagnosis is

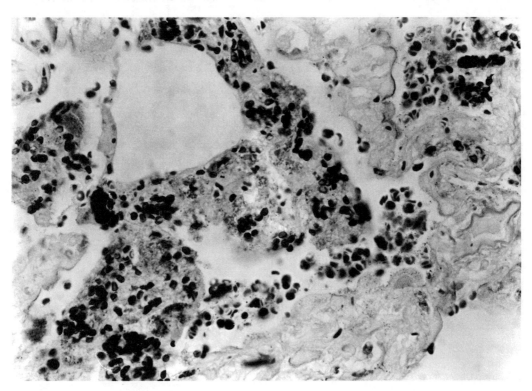

(A) atypical mycobacterial infection
(B) cytomegalovirus (CMV) pneumonitis
(C) nocardial abscess
(D) pneumocystis pneumonia
(E) legionnaires' disease

32. A 24-year-old black woman presented with chest pain; her chest radiograph revealed mediastinal lymphadenopathy. A lymph node biopsy from the anterior mediastinum was obtained by mediastinoscopy, and the tissue sample is portrayed in the photomicrograph below. The correct diagnosis is

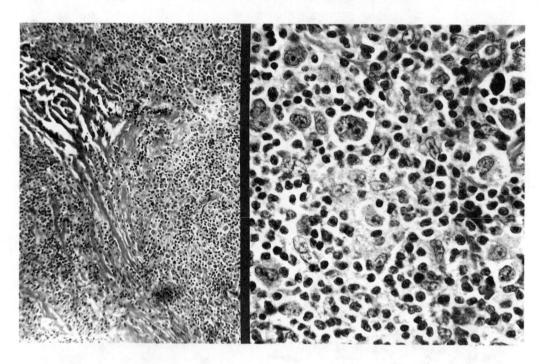

(A) sarcoidosis
(B) thymoma
(C) sclerosing mediastinitis
(D) Hodgkin's disease

33. Which of the following statements regarding the proximal tubular epithelium illustrated below is most likely to be correct?

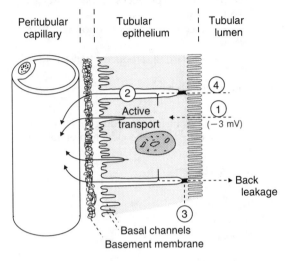

Peritubular capillary | Tubular epithelium | Tubular lumen

(A) The ion whose movement is depicted in (*1*) is Na$^+$

(B) The process depicted at site (*2*) is aldosterone-sensitive

(C) The cell is impermeable to water because of the tight junctions shown in (*3*)

(D) The process depicted at site (*4*) is affected by antidiuretic hormone (ADH)

(E) The intracellular potential is similar to the tubular lumen potential (-3 mV)

34. Of the following statements regarding thoracic outlet syndrome, which one is true?

(A) It results from an irregularly shaped first thoracic rib

(B) Compression of the left phrenic nerve may occur

(C) Numbness and tingling occur along a median nerve distribution

(D) Compression of the subclavian artery may occur

35. Glucose stimulation of beta cells in the endocrine pancreas subsequently causes

(A) enhancement of gluconeogenesis in the liver

(B) increased glycogenolysis by the liver

(C) stimulation of the release of glucagon

(D) decreased oxidation of amino acids in the liver

36. Each of the following statements concerning intercostal nerves is true EXCEPT that

(A) they are the anterior rami of the 12 thoracic spinal nerves

(B) they are connected to the sympathetic trunk by rami communicans

(C) the first intercostal nerve is joined to the brachial plexus

(D) they supply the anterior abdominal muscles

(E) they supply the parietal pleura

37. A man is brought to the emergency room after being beaten with a baseball bat. He received one blow to the head, which did not fracture the skull. At which of the following locations would a blow cause the LEAST amount of damage to the brain, assuming that all blows were delivered with equal force?

(A) The side of the head

(B) The front of the head

(C) The back of the head

(D) A glancing blow to the back of the head

Questions 38–39

A 55-year-old patient presents with weakness, weight loss, and bone pain of 3-months duration. Head x-rays show many well-demarcated osteolytic lesions.

38. All of the following symptoms would help to confirm the diagnosis of this disease EXCEPT

(A) the presence of monoclonal proteins weighing 55,000 daltons in the serum and urine

(B) a history of recurrent bacterial infections

(C) a spike in a particular isotype region in the electrophoretic pattern of serum proteins

(D) the presence of Bence Jones protein in the serum or urine

39. In approximately 55% of patients presenting with multiple myeloma, the major membrane-bound carrier protein, or monoclonal protein, would be

(A) immunoglobulin M (IgM)

(B) IgD

(C) IgE

(D) IgA

(E) IgG

40. Monitoring aminoglycoside serum levels is requisite for the systemic use of the drugs because

(A) they are extensively metabolized by hepatic enzymes

(B) they are rapidly eliminated

(C) they can cause severe hypersensitivity reactions

(D) their therapeutic index is low, and toxicity is easily manifest

(E) they rapidly cross the blood–brain barrier

41. Tamoxifen can control the growth of some forms of female breast cancer by

(A) inhibiting estrogen synthesis

(B) inhibiting androgen-induced DNA transcription

(C) competing for estrogen receptors

(D) inhibiting the secretion of luteinizing hormone (LH)

(E) stimulating nuclear transcription

42. Propranolol (a β-blocker) may be used with nitroglycerin (glyceryl trinitrate; GTN) in concurrent therapy for typical (exertional) angina because propranolol

(A) is a potent vasodilator of coronary arteries

(B) increases conduction in the atria and atrioventricular node

(C) blocks the reflex tachycardia that occurs with the use of GTN

(D) dilates constricted airways

(E) is positively inotropic

43. Phenytoin (Dilantin) is effective in most forms of epilepsy (with the exception of absence seizures) because it

(A) directly binds to chloride channels in the central nervous system (CNS)

(B) enhances the inhibitory actions of γ-aminobutyric acid (GABA) at its receptor in the CNS

(C) affects Na^+ conductance in neurons via voltage-sensitive Na^+-channel inhibition

(D) is usually started concurrently with phenobarbital therapy

44. Which one of the following statements concerning the synthesis of different types of RNA molecules in eukaryotic cells is true?

(A) RNA polymerase I produces mainly messenger RNA (mRNA)

(B) RNA polymerase III produces ribosomal RNA (rRNA)

(C) RNA polymerase II produces transfer RNA (tRNA)

(D) None of the above

45. Which one of the following drugs or chemicals has been associated with the induction of aplastic anemia?

(A) Acetaminophen

(B) Methyldopa

(C) Benzene

(D) Penicillin

(E) Thiouracil

46. A monoclonal antibody (immunoglobulin G; IgG) that neutralizes endotoxin has been produced. This antibody has tremendous therapeutic potential for patients suffering septic shock from endotoxemia, and it might be useful in treating patients who have which one of the following diseases?

(A) Pulmonary anthrax

(B) Whooping cough

(C) Cholera

(D) Leprosy

(E) Bubonic plague

47. Which of the following proteins bind to penicillin?

(A) Alanine racemase

(B) 30S Ribosomes

(C) Peptidoglycan

(D) Porin

(E) Transpeptidase

48. All of the following statements concerning mammalian chromosomes are true EXCEPT

(A) DNase I can be used to treat chromosomes to determine inactive regions of DNA

(B) approximately 7% of the sequences contained in the eukaryotic genome are ever copied into RNA

(C) heterochromatin is a term used for inactive DNA, and euchromatin is a term used for those regions of DNA that are transcriptionally active

(D) in higher eukaryotic genomes, cytosine is methylated at CG islands in inactive segments of DNA

49. A medical student received a deep laceration in an altercation at a party. He reports having had a DTP (diphtheria-tetanus-pertussis) series in childhood. The most appropriate treatment would be

(A) injection of human tetanus immunoglobulin G (IgG)

(B) injection of equine tetanus IgG

(C) intravenous administration of an aminoglycoside

(D) injection of tetanus toxoid

50. Which of the following statements concerning acetylsalicylic acid (aspirin), the prototype of a group of nonsteroidal anti-inflammatory agents that are also analgesic and antipyretic, is correct?

(A) Aspirin is a potent lipoxygenase inhibitor

(B) The major adverse effect of aspirin is gastrointestinal bleeding

(C) Aspirin can reduce normal body temperature

(D) Aspirin is a competitive inhibitor of platelet cyclooxygenase

51. Which one of the following statements concerning messenger RNA (mRNA) splicing is true?

(A) Alternate splicing, producing two different mRNA molecules from the same gene, is a common occurrence in most mammalian genes

(B) Spliceosomes are collections of small nuclear ribonucleoproteins (snRNPs) located near ribosomes on the rough endoplasmic reticulum

(C) U1 snRNP binds to a nucleotide segment on the 5' end of the intron to be spliced

(D) Spliceosomes recognize splicing sites by the large 50–80 base-pair sequences on the 5' and 3' regions of introns

52. The most common tumor of the appendix, which is pictured below, is

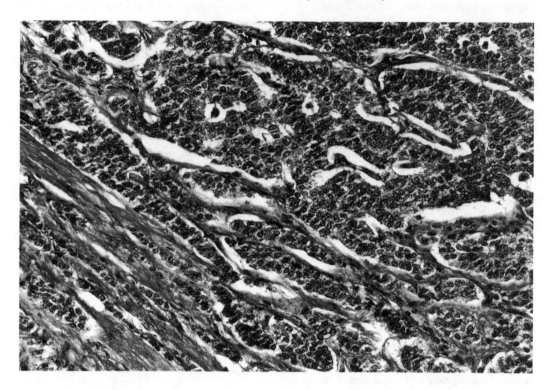

(A) a carcinoid tumor
(B) an adenocarcinoma
(C) a mucocele
(D) an inflammatory pseudotumor

53. Each of the following enzymes is essential for protecting red blood cells from the hydrogen peroxide generated in vivo EXCEPT

(A) glutathione peroxidase
(B) 6-phosphogluconate dehydrogenase
(C) catalase
(D) transketolase
(E) glutathione reductase

54. All of the following statements concerning the Arthus reaction are true EXCEPT

(A) it usually requires large amounts of antibody and antigen
(B) it results in localized rupture of vessel walls followed by tissue necrosis
(C) neutrophils and platelets are present at the site of the reaction
(D) it is the most common type III reaction seen in humans

55. Zidovudine (ZDV) [formerly known as azido-thymidine (AZT)] has all of the following properties EXCEPT

(A) ZDV reduces the chances of progression to AIDS in asymptomatic human immunodeficiency virus (HIV)–infected subjects
(B) ZDV improves the clinical symptoms of immunologic function, survival period, and quality of life of advanced AIDS patients
(C) ZDV is very toxic to bone marrow
(D) ZDV is effective only in the treatment of patients with advanced AIDS
(E) prolonged treatment with ZDV (1–3 years) results in resistance to this drug

56. All of the following mediators released during mast cell activation cause an increase of vascular permeability EXCEPT

(A) histamine

(B) eosinophil chemotactic factor (ECF)

(C) serotonin

(D) slow-reacting substance of anaphylaxis

57. Major risk factors for the development of chronic obstructive pulmonary disease (COPD) include all of the following EXCEPT

(A) smoking

(B) air pollution

(C) occupational exposure to irritant gases and particles

(D) α_1-antitrypsin deficiency

(E) intravenous drug abuse

58. Which one of the following conditions would result in a negative nitrogen balance?

(A) Consumption of dietary proteins that are deficient in glycine

(B) Normal intake of dietary protein accompanied by defective cholecystokinin–pancreozymin (CCK-PZ) production

(C) Nitrogen consumption that exceeds nitrogen excretion

(D) A tyrosine supplement in the diet of a child with phenylketonuria (PKU)

(E) A 50% reduction in the hydrochloric acid (HCl) content of gastric juice

59. Characteristics of Duchenne muscular dystrophy (DMD) include all of the following EXCEPT

(A) decreased amounts of dystrophin in affected muscles

(B) hypertrophy of affected muscle groups

(C) autosomal dominant inheritance via mutated chromosome 20

(D) one-third of the cases resulting from spontaneous mutation

(E) sarcomere hypercontraction and contraction band formation

60. A young child develops pharyngitis, a fever, and a rash. β-Hemolytic, gram-positive cocci in chains are isolated from the throat and are found to be catalase-negative. All of the following statements about the virulence factors of this pathogen are true EXCEPT

(A) hemolysis results from production of extracellular hemolysins

(B) the organism produces membrane-bound protein (M protein), which has antiphagocytic properties

(C) the organism produces lipoteichoic acid, which is necessary for attachment to mucosa

(D) the organism is not encapsulated

(E) the rash is produced by a toxin distinct from the hemolysins

61. Translation of a synthetic polyribonucleotide containing the repeating sequence CAA in a cell-free protein synthesizing system produced three homopolypeptides: polyglutamine, polyasparagine, and polythreonine. If the codons for glutamine and asparagine are CAA and AAC, respectively, which of the following triplets is a codon for threonine?

(A) AAC

(B) CAA

(C) CAC

(D) CCA

(E) ACA

Questions 62–63

It is hypothesized that nocturnal body temperatures are linearly related to body weight in 60- to 70-year-old women. Nursing records are reviewed for weights in kilograms and 4 A.M. temperatures in degrees Celsius.

62. These variables are considered to be

(A) continuous
(B) nonparametric
(C) constants
(D) reciprocal
(E) outliers

63. The null hypothesis for the study question described would state that there is

(A) an expected correlation between body weight and temperature
(B) an effect of aging on temperatures in obese elderly women
(C) no relationship between temperature and body weight
(D) an inverse relationship between body weight and nocturnal temperature
(E) a probability ($P < 0.05$) that body weight is related to nocturnal temperature

64. *Pseudomonas aeruginosa, Staphylococcus aureus,* and *Serratia marcescens* all produce which one of the following substances?

(A) Endotoxins
(B) Enterotoxins
(C) Lipoteichoic acids
(D) Mycolic acids
(E) Pigments

65. Resistance to phagocytosis is among the most important properties for virulence of many bacteria. *Mycobacterium tuberculosis* is very resistant to phagocytic killing and actually grows in macrophages. The successful antiphagocytic strategy employed by *M. tuberculosis* clearly involves which one of the following mechanisms?

(A) Production of protein exotoxins to kill or impair the phagocyte
(B) Prevention of phagosome–lysosome fusion
(C) Elaboration of immunoglobulin A (IgA) protease
(D) Production of the antiphagocytic polysaccharide capsule
(E) Escape from the phagolysosome into the cytoplasm

66. Injection of a pharmacologically effective amount of an antimuscarinic agent, like atropine, may

(A) increase bronchial glandular secretions
(B) increase heart rate
(C) cause paralysis in some skeletal muscles
(D) constrict the pupil
(E) promote sweating

67. G proteins are involved with various cellular signaling pathways and are known to hydrolyze

(A) adenosine triphosphate (ATP)
(B) guanosine triphosphate (GTP)
(C) adenosine diphosphate (ADP)
(D) guanosine diphosphate (GDP)
(E) adenosine monophosphate (AMP)

68. A peripheral lung nodule was resected from a 50-year-old man. The tumor, pictured below, is best classified as

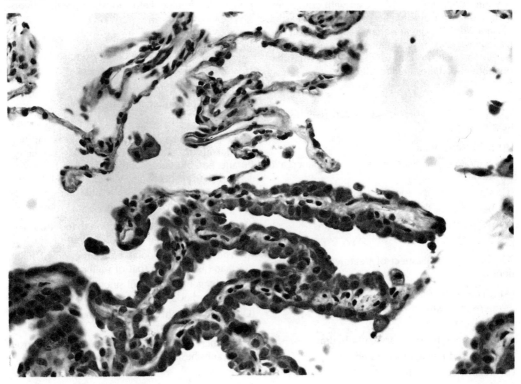

(A) small cell carcinoma

(B) undifferentiated large cell carcinoma

(C) adenoid cystic carcinoma

(D) bronchioloalveolar carcinoma

(E) diffuse large cell lymphoma

69. Cushing's syndrome is a complex array of symptoms that are due to excess glucocorticoid levels. All of the following statements about Cushing's syndrome are correct EXCEPT

(A) the disease may be associated with an adenoma of the pituitary corticotropes

(B) the disease may be secondary to abnormal hypothalamic function with excessive release of corticotropin releasing factor (CRF)

(C) the disease may be due to ectopic adrenocorticotropic hormone (ACTH) synthesis

(D) some aspects of the syndrome may be due to long-term therapy with glucocorticoids

(E) increased long bone length is common in patients prior to puberty

70. A lymph node removed from a 32-year-old man shows diffuse large cell lymphoma. Which of the following clinical scenarios most likely characterizes this patient?

(A) Disseminated disease at presentation; prolonged survival eventually succumbing to lymphoma or its complications

(B) Rapid development of circulating immature blasts, requiring aggressive cytotoxic therapy

(C) Greater than 90% chance of being alive 10 years after diagnosis

(D) Rapid death if therapy is unsuccessful; approximately 50% chance for long-term survival if therapy achieves complete response

(E) Spontaneous remission in 20% of patients

Questions 71–75

A young adult visits his physician with complaints of polyuria and unexplained weight loss. Fasting plasma glucose is greater than 140 mg/dl (on two occasions), and an oral glucose tolerance test is consistent with a diagnosis of type I insulin-dependent diabetes mellitus (IDDM).

71. The likely histologic site underlying this patient's disorder is

(A) pancreatic acini
(B) zymogen-containing cells of the pancreatic acinus
(C) alpha cell of the islets of Langerhans
(D) beta cells of the islets of Langerhans
(E) delta cells of the islets of Langerhans

72. An important aspect of treatment in this patient is

(A) a single daily injection of an insulin zinc suspension (Lente insulin)
(B) glipizide
(C) abstinence from dietary carbohydrates
(D) increased intake of saturated fats
(E) avoidance of exercise

73. An endogenous hormone that tends to decrease circulating blood glucose is

(A) glucagon
(B) growth hormone (GH)
(C) somatostatin
(D) epinephrine
(E) thyroid hormone

74. In spite of vigorous therapy, all of the following are potential chronic complications of IDDM EXCEPT

(A) intercapillary glomerulosclerosis
(B) proliferative retinopathy
(C) atherosclerosis
(D) peripheral polyneuropathy
(E) pulmonary hypertension

75. The patient is brought to the emergency room in a coma. An important clue suggesting that the coma is the result of ketoacidosis rather than hypoglycemia is

(A) history of a missed meal
(B) history of unusual vigorous exercise
(C) rapid, deep ventilatory pattern
(D) profuse sweating
(E) normal hydration status

76. Halothane has blood:gas and oil:gas partition coefficients of 2.4 and 220, respectively. Methoxyflurane has blood:gas and oil:gas coefficients of 13 and 950, respectively. Which of the following statements regarding these volatile anesthetics is correct?

(A) Both result in faster induction than nitrous oxide (blood:gas partition coefficient of 0.47)
(B) The minimal alveolar concentration of halothane is less than that of methoxyflurane
(C) Both agents are useful since they do not have any cardiodepressant effects
(D) Recovery from methoxyflurane is faster than that from halothane
(E) An increase in ventilatory rate makes the onset of anesthesia more rapid for either agent

77. All of the following statements about protein synthesis are true EXCEPT

(A) the activated form of an amino acid is called aminoacyl transfer RNA (tRNA)
(B) the addition of aminoacyl tRNA to the growing peptide chain and subsequent translocation is an energy-requiring process
(C) the formation of the peptide bond is catalyzed by peptidyltransferase
(D) synthesis occurs in the mitochondria as well as in the cytoplasm of cells
(E) synthesis can occur in the absence of RNA

78. Restriction enzymes have which one of the following characteristics? They

(A) can only cleave circular DNA
(B) generate either staggered (sticky) or blunt ends upon cleaving DNA
(C) cleave different DNAs randomly
(D) can cleave different DNAs only once
(E) can cleave both DNA and RNA

79. A chronically ill 43-year-old patient with a relapse of multiple sclerosis has been in the hospital for 4 weeks. He has angered the nurses by being very demanding, including calling them "every 5 minutes" for minor reasons and complaining that they do not respond promptly. To remedy this situation, the physician must

(A) instruct the patient to behave better

(B) order a sedating medication

(C) arrange for the nurses to visit the patient for 3 minutes every hour

(D) warn the patient that he will be transferred to another hospital if he does not straighten out

80. Each statement below concerning osteoclasts is true EXCEPT that they

(A) are found in Howship's lacuna

(B) resorb bone

(C) are stimulated by calcitonin

(D) are multinucleated

(E) help remodel bone

81. A 74-year-old man presents with hypertension, diabetes mellitus with retinopathy, and chronic obstructive pulmonary disease (COPD). He admits to drinking four bottles of beer a day. He has been living alone for the past year since his wife died. His primary care physician should be especially and immediately concerned about the risk of

(A) renal insufficiency

(B) silent myocardial infarction

(C) suicide

(D) peripheral neuropathy

(E) pneumonia

82. Asymptomatic bacteriuria is noted in a 35-year-old pregnant woman in her second trimester. Five years ago, during her first pregnancy, she presented with acute pyelonephritis, which required hospitalization and parenteral antibacterial therapy. Since then, recurrent sexual intercourse–related urinary tract infections have been prevented by a single dose of nitrofurantoin after coitus. All of the following agents would be contraindicated for this patient during the remainder of her pregnancy for prevention of acute pyelonephritis EXCEPT

(A) trimethoprim/sulfamethoxazole

(B) minocycline

(C) amoxicillin

(D) gentamicin

83. The graph below measures the number of viable bacterial cells in a control culture and cultures of exponentially growing cells to which antibiotics were added at the point indicated by the *arrow*. The antibiotic added to the culture to produce *curve A* was which one of the following?

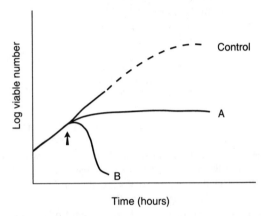

(A) Polymyxin B

(B) Cephalothin

(C) Chloramphenicol

(D) Methicillin

(E) Vancomycin

84. According to the Henderson-Hasselbalch equation:

$$pH = 6.1 + \log [HCO_3^-]/0.03 \times P_{CO_2}$$

The apparent dissociation constant, pK′, in blood is 6.1; and the solubility constant for CO_2 in plasma at 38° C is 0.03 mmol/L/mm Hg. If a patient has a plasma $[HCO_3^-]$ of 37 mmol/L and arterial P_{CO_2} of 60 mm Hg, then the patient is most likely to have (recall log 10 = 1; log 20 = 1.3; log 30 = 1.5; normal values of $[HCO_3^-]$ = 25 mmol/L; P_{CO_2} = 40 mm Hg)

(A) respiratory alkalosis

(B) respiratory acidosis

(C) fully compensated respiratory acidosis

(D) metabolic alkalosis

(E) metabolic acidosis

85. Thymomas are associated with all of the following diseases EXCEPT

(A) myasthenia gravis

(B) systemic lupus erythematosus

(C) hypogammaglobulinemia

(D) Graves' disease

(E) neutrophil agranulocytosis

(F) polymyositis

86. The ability of erythrocytes to pump Na^+ from the cytoplasm into the plasma compartment would be compromised most directly by a total deficiency of

(A) stearoyl coenzyme A (CoA) desaturase
(B) diphosphoglycerate kinase
(C) pyruvate carboxylase
(D) glucose 6-phosphatase
(E) malate dehydrogenase

87. All of the following statements concerning the human immunodeficiency virus (HIV) are true EXCEPT that

(A) the virus can infect T cells, macrophages, and any other cell type with a CD4 receptor
(B) viral infection can spread between cells without the involvement of free virus
(C) the viral infection process involves endocytosis of the HIV particle into the cell
(D) replication of the viral nucleic acid occurs in the nucleus

88. A total of 25 hypertensive patients are followed over a 2-week period for the effects of a diuretic drug on K^+ concentrations. The statistical test used to compare the K^+ serum levels before and after medication is most likely to be

(A) discriminant analysis
(B) paired t-test
(C) regression analysis
(D) chi-squared test
(E) Pearson correlation

89. For antibiotic therapy, it is useful to understand both the action of the prescribed antibiotic and the pathogenesis of the bacteria responsible for a patient's infection. For example, the aminoglycoside antibiotic gentamicin does not enter mammalian cells and, therefore, is ineffective against intracellular pathogens. Considering only this information, gentamicin is effective against all of the following infections EXCEPT

(A) *Hemophilus influenzae* type B epiglottitis
(B) *Pseudomonas aeruginosa* burn infections
(C) *Klebsiella pneumoniae* respiratory infections
(D) *Escherichia coli* urinary tract infections
(E) *Chlamydia trachomatis* infections

Questions 90–91

A 22-year-old male college student visits the student health service complaining of extreme fatigue, sore throat, difficulty concentrating, and fever to 39° C over the last week. Physical examination is unremarkable except for mild lymph node enlargement in axillary, cervical, and inguinal regions and a palpable spleen tip. A blood count shows hemoglobin of 10 g/dl, platelets of 105,000/μl, and white cell count of 22,000/μl with 60% lymphoid cells. The laboratory blood profile also shows an absolute red cell count of 2.3×10^6/μl, mean red cell volume of 125 femtoliters (fl), and mean cell hemoglobin concentration of 43 g/dl.

90. What is the most likely diagnosis for this patient?

(A) Infectious lymphocytosis
(B) *Bordetella pertussis* infection
(C) Cytomegalovirus (CMV) mononucleosis syndrome
(D) Mononucleosis secondary to Epstein-Barr virus (EBV) infection (infectious mononucleosis)
(E) Mononucleosis secondary to *Toxoplasma gondii* infection

91. Which of the following is the most likely etiology for this patient's anemia (Hb 10 g/dl)?

(A) Immune-mediated
(B) Compromise of erythroid production secondary to EBV infection of bone marrow precursors
(C) Virus-associated hemophagocytic syndrome
(D) Slow gastrointestinal blood loss since the start of illness due to thrombocytopenia
(E) Disseminated intravascular coagulation (DIC)

92. The eclipse phase of the virus replication cycle has which one of the following characteristics? It

(A) is defined as that time period after which the first virus particles are assembled
(B) denotes the time between virus entry into the cell and the time virus particles appear extracellularly
(C) is that part of the replication cycle during which virus particles cannot be recovered from the infected cells
(D) is comparable to the metaphase portion of mitosis

93. Light microscopy requires the use of special techniques, such as stains, to visualize cells and cell components. Which of the following cellular components can be visualized after staining for catalase?

(A) Golgi complex

(B) Lysosomes

(C) Rough endoplasmic reticulum

(D) Smooth endoplasmic reticulum

(E) Peroxisomes

94. Dinitrochlorobenzene was applied to a patient's skin over a 1-cm^2 area on the right forearm. About 2 weeks later, a pruritic rash occurred at the site. It can be concluded that

(A) the patient lacks all T-cell–mediated immune function

(B) the patient suffers from DiGeorge syndrome

(C) the reaction would require an additional 2 weeks to develop on subsequent exposure to dinitrochlorobenzene

(D) the reaction observed was most likely caused by CD4$^+$ T cells

Questions 95–97

An ophthalmologic examination of a 60-year-old man complaining of vision problems reveals increased intraocular pressure (25 mm Hg) with optic disk changes and visual field defects. These findings strongly suggest primary open-angle glaucoma for which pharmacotherapy is considered.

95. The underlying cause of the patient's condition is a decreased outflow facility of the aqueous humor. A primary anatomic structure involved with the histopathologic changes that account for this problem is the

(A) conjunctiva

(B) cornea

(C) canal of Schlemm

(D) ciliary process

(E) choroidal vessel

96. Pharmacotherapy for the above patient is initially designed to open trabecular meshwork by contracting the ciliary muscle. A useful agent for this purpose is

(A) atropine

(B) succinylcholine

(C) pilocarpine

(D) dexamethasone

(E) tubocurarine

97. After the initial pharmacotherapy fails, the patient is switched to an anticholinesterase agent, echothiophate. Absorption of this agent from the eye may be associated with which of the following adverse systemic effects?

(A) Tachycardia

(B) Urinary retention

(C) Decrease in gastrointesinal motility

(D) Bronchoconstriction

(E) Inappropriate decrease in sweating

98. The peripheral nerve tumor pictured below is best classified as a

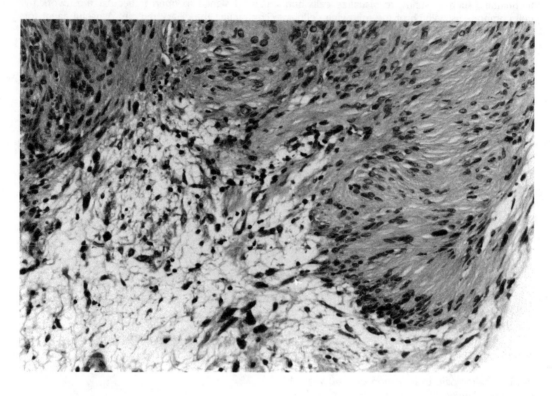

(A) neurofibroma

(B) traumatic neuroma

(C) neurilemoma

(D) triton tumor

99. All of the following statements concerning the response of immunoglobulins to viruses in vivo are true EXCEPT they

(A) displace attached viruses from the host cell

(B) inhibit the action of viral enzymes

(C) induce complement-mediated lysis of infected host cells

(D) retard the infectivity of viruses for host cells

100. Triglycerides are neutral fats of animals and food plants; they make up about 90% of the dietary intake of fats. An important step in their digestive fate in the gastrointestinal tract is

(A) significant hydrolysis by gastric lipases

(B) breakdown by biliary enzymes

(C) formation of fatty acids and monoglyceride by pancreatic lipase

(D) active transport of fatty acid products in the intestinal brush border

101. Cholesterol biosynthesis occurs in the cytosol of many cells of the body, primarily in the liver, and entails all of the following steps EXCEPT it

(A) forms lanosterol from squalene and then converts it to cholesterol

(B) requires reduced nicotinamide-adenine dinucleotide phosphate (NADPH) as a source of reducing equivalents

(C) forms 3-hydroxy-3-methylglutaryl coenzyme A (HMG CoA) from acetoacetyl CoA

(D) forms squalene from isoprenoid units

(E) uses HMG CoA reductase for catalysis of HMG CoA to mevinolin

102. Which of the tracts listed below is thought to cross to the opposite side of the central nervous system (CNS) twice as its fibers traverse the spinal cord, brain stem, and higher structures?

(A) The anterior spinocerebellar tract, which conveys unconscious sensory information from joints, tendons, and muscles

(B) The spinal thalamic tract, which conveys conscious sensory information of pain and temperature

(C) The cuneocerebellar tract, which conveys conscious muscle and joint sensory information

(D) The vestibulospinal tract, which conveys efferent fibers

103. A 29-year-old white woman comes to the physician's office stating that she recently discovered a gap in her memory of 2 hours. She tells the physician that her friends informed her that she has been acting inappropriately. Suddenly the patient becomes confused but remains docile. She asks the physician from where the overwhelming smell of rotten food is emanating. The patient most likely suffers from

(A) Klüver-Bucy syndrome of the temporal lobes

(B) temporal lobe epilepsy

(C) jacksonian epileptic seizures

(D) petit mal seizures

104. A 5-year-old child in Bangladesh drinks untreated river water and develops cholera. Which of the following scenarios is most likely to occur?

(A) Recovery following treatment is slow because *Vibrio cholerae* causes chronic intracellular infections

(B) Microscopic examination of stools reveals leukocytes

(C) Disease symptoms arise due to cholera toxin-mediated elevation in cyclic adenosine monophosphate (cAMP) levels in intestinal cells

(D) *V. cholerae* attaches to the dental flora

105. Angiotensin-converting enzyme (ACE) hydrolyzes angiotensin I to angiotensin II. Possible explanations as to why inhibition of this enzyme with specific peptide inhibitors (i.e., captopril) reduces blood pressure in some subjects include all of the following EXCEPT

(A) decreased production of a vasoconstrictor (angiotensin II)

(B) increased synthesis and release of aldosterone

(C) centrally mediated decrease in water intake

(D) inhibition of synaptic transmission in peripheral sympathetic nervous system

106. Centrioles are replicated in which phase of the cell cycle?

(A) G_0 phase
(B) G_1 phase
(C) S phase
(D) G_2 phase
(E) M phase

107. Which one of the following statements about energy storage and transfer is true?

(A) Adenosine triphosphate (ATP) can be synthesized from adenosine diphosphate (ADP) by phosphate transfer from 3-phosphoglycerate

(B) Phosphocreatine is an important energy source for muscle tissues

(C) Reactions that have a $K_{eq} > 1$ have a positive $\Delta G°$

(D) When ATP is hydrolyzed to adenosine monophosphate (AMP) and inorganic pyrophosphate (PP_i), the reaction is endergonic and will proceed spontaneously

(E) The energy of hydrolysis for phosphoenolpyruvate is less than that for pyrophosphate

108. The extraction of β-hydroxybutyrate from blood and its oxidation to carbon dioxide and water requires the participation of

(A) β-hydroxybutyrate dehydrogenase and 3-hydroxy-3-methylglutaryl coenzyme A (HMG CoA) lyase

(B) acetoacetate thiokinase and β-hydroxybutyrate dehydrogenase

(C) HMG CoA synthase and thiolase

(D) short-chain fatty acetyl CoA dehydrogenase and thiolase

(E) succinyl CoA: acetoacetate acyltransferase and HMG CoA lyase

Questions 109–111

A 43-year-old man who is being treated with hydrochlorothiazide for control of mild edema presents to the physician complaining of malaise, fatigue, muscular weakness, and muscle cramps. Blood tests reveal elevated creatinine with an even greater elevation in blood urea nitrogen, high blood urate, and altered blood electrolytes.

109. What is the primary anatomic site of action of hydrochlorothiazide?

(A) Proximal tubules

(B) Early distal tubules

(C) Late distal tubules

(D) Thick ascending limb of the loop of Henle

(E) Collecting ducts

110. The patient's complaints most likely reflect the most serious adverse effect of diuretic therapy, which is

(A) hyperglycemia

(B) hyperuricemia

(C) drug hypersensitivity

(D) hyperkalemia

(E) hypokalemia

111. To correct this patient's problem, the physician must consider all of the following therapeutic choices EXCEPT

(A) K^+ supplementation

(B) digitalis

(C) spironolactone

(D) reduced dosage of hydrochlorothiazide

(E) amiloride

112. A 60-year-old woman is brought to the hospital because of fever and confusion. One week ago, she received chemotherapy for lymphoma. In the emergency room, she is noted to have rapid breathing, cool, clammy skin, and a blood pressure of 70/40. Complete blood count shows a white blood cell count of $200/\mu l$. Gram stains of urine and sputum are negative. Which of the following empiric therapies would be most appropriate for this patient?

(A) Gentamicin

(B) Amikacin

(C) Chloramphenicol–gentamicin

(D) Piperacillin–gentamicin

113. An adolescent patient attends weekly individual, psychodynamic psychotherapy sessions. When he begins to feel too close to and dependent on the psychiatrist, he often misses a scheduled appointment. This behavior is an example of

(A) acting out

(B) antisocial personality

(C) repression

(D) suppression

(E) identification with the aggressor

114. Which of the statements below concerning the disaccharide pictured below is most accurate? It

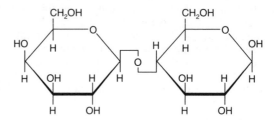

(A) yields a negative result in the Fehling-Benedict reducing sugar test

(B) is cleaved by isomaltose

(C) is a β-galactoside

(D) is digested and absorbed by a lactase-deficient child

(E) is a good source of calories for a 2-week-old child with galactosemia

115. A 42-year-old woman with breast cancer was treated with irradiation and currently is receiving chemotherapy. She complained of some left-sided chest pain, which was determined not to be of cardiac origin. On the fourth day, several vesicles appeared on her left thorax, following a rib in distribution; she also had several smaller vesicles at other sites (scalp, leg, forearm). Her physician diagnosed varicella-zoster virus (VZV) infection and started treatment with acyclovir. Which one of the following statements best describes the VZV in this case?

(A) Thymidine kinase-negative VZV mutants are likely to render the treatment ineffective

(B) The initial exposure to VZV in childhood could not have led to viral latency in the dorsal ganglia

(C) The lesions outside the dermatomal distribution are likely explained by depressed cell-mediated immunity

116. A 62-year-old woman died of congestive heart failure due to severe mitral stenosis. At autopsy, sections of the heart revealed the lesions shown in the photomicrograph below. This suggests a previous history of which one of the following conditions?

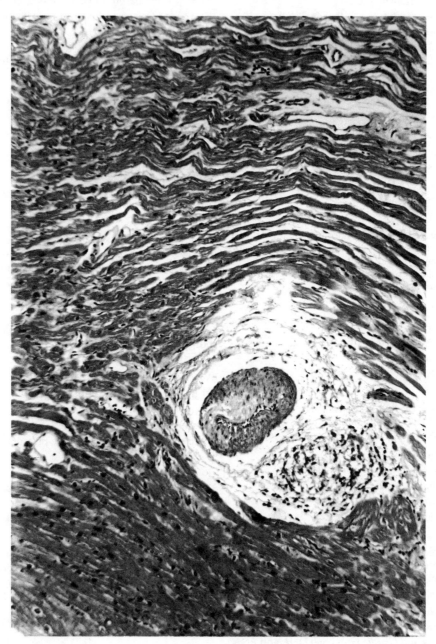

(A) Amyloidosis

(B) Rheumatic fever

(C) Polyarteritis nodosa

(D) Myocardial infarction

117. Which of the following tests is the major projective instrument of personality assessment?

(A) Rorschach inkblot test
(B) Minnesota Multiphasic Personality Inventory
(C) Thematic apperception test
(D) Sentence completion test
(E) Projective drawings

118. All of the following substances readily diffuse through cell membranes EXCEPT

(A) oxygen
(B) carbon dioxide
(C) glucose
(D) water
(E) nitrogen

119. The S_3 heart sound is normally heard only in children or young, thin-chested adults. An accentuated S_3 heart sound can sometimes be heard in either children or adults with all of the following pathologies EXCEPT

(A) mitral regurgitation
(B) patent ductus arteriosus
(C) left ventricular failure
(D) pulmonary stenosis
(E) ventricular septal defects

120. Proof of the presence of active disease caused by *Mycobacterium tuberculosis* is provided by which one of the following diagnostic measures?

(A) The tuberculin test
(B) Clinical findings (e.g., weight loss, night sweats, cough, low-grade fever)
(C) Finding acid-fast organisms in sputum
(D) Isolation of *M. tuberculosis*

121. A fecal specimen is cultured from a person with diarrhea, and *Shigella dysenteriae* and *Giardia lamblia* are isolated. All of the following statements about *Shigella* and *Giardia* are true EXCEPT

(A) *Shigella* has a peptidoglycan-containing cell wall but *G. lamblia* does not
(B) *Shigella* and *Giardia* both have DNA and RNA
(C) *Shigella* and *Giardia* both have sterol-containing plasma membranes
(D) *Shigella* has a lipopolysaccharide but *Giardia* does not
(E) *Shigella* has 70S ribosomes but *Giardia* has 80S ribosomes

122. All of the following statements about enzymes are true EXCEPT that

(A) V_{max} is a measure of catalytic efficiency
(B) K_m is a measure of the enzyme's affinity for the substrate
(C) formation of the substrate complex results in rearrangement of specific functional groups of the enzyme
(D) the reaction rate is accelerated by increasing the activation energy
(E) they frequently use ionizable amino acid side chains as general acids and bases in catalysis

123. Several workers at a chemical manufacturing facility were referred to a physician for evaluation of connective tissue neoplasms. This physician could expect to find

(A) antigenic cross-reactivity between tumors
(B) distinct antigenic specificity for each tumor
(C) antigenic cross-reactivity between these tumors and those induced by ultraviolet light
(D) distinct antigenic specificity for different cells from the same tumor

124. Adult respiratory distress syndrome (ARDS) shows all of the following morphologic signs EXCEPT

(A) pulmonary edema
(B) hyaline membrane formation
(C) proliferation of type II pneumocytes
(D) alveolar wall damage
(E) decreased permeability of the pulmonary capillary endothelium

125. Type II pneumocytes have all of the following characteristics EXCEPT

(A) they elaborate pulmonary surfactant
(B) they exhibit surface microvilli
(C) they make up most of the alveolar surface area
(D) they contain osmiophilic lamellar bodies
(E) defects in these cells contribute to infant and adult respiratory distress

126. Hodgkin's lymphoma can be distinguished from other forms of lymphoma by the presence of

(A) Reed-Sternberg cells
(B) the Philadelphia chromosome
(C) Auer rods
(D) decreased quantities of leukocyte alkaline phosphatase

127. All of the following intracellular substances are second messengers in mammalian cells EXCEPT

(A) inositol 1,4,5-triphosphate (IP_3)
(B) cyclic adenosine monophosphate (cAMP)
(C) Ca^{2+}
(D) diacylglycerol (DAG)
(E) c-*fos*

128. An 86-year-old man has diminished vibratory sensation at the knees and toes, although his reflexes are intact, temperature sensation is normal, and he feels well, aside from headaches. What is the most likely explanation?

(A) Peripheral neuropathy
(B) Normal age-related change
(C) Spinal cord lesion
(D) Small strokes
(E) Brain or brain stem tumor

129. Embolism of a cerebral artery most commonly occurs from all of the following situations EXCEPT

(A) atheromatous plaques of the vertebral artery
(B) atheromatous plaques of the internal carotid artery
(C) endocarditis of the mitral valve
(D) atheromatous plaques of the abdominal aorta

130. The pressor response to an indirect-acting sympathomimetic agent, such as amphetamine, is

(A) associated with marked tolerance (tachyphylaxis)
(B) decreased in the presence of a monoamine oxidase (MAO) inhibitor
(C) potentiated by an uptake 1 inhibitor, such as imipramine
(D) potentiated by pretreatment with reserpine
(E) related to its direct effects on postsynaptic receptors

131. The introduction of foreign DNA into bacteria is an important tool in molecular biology. Which of the following statements concerning nucleic acid transfer is true?

(A) Transformation is the technique whereby a bacteriophage is used to introduce DNA into a bacteria
(B) Transduction is the technique whereby "competent" bacterial cells are suspended in a solution of calcium chloride and DNA
(C) The most common DNA used in transformation is plasmid DNA
(D) Conjugation is the technique whereby a bacteriophage is used to introduce DNA into a bacteria

Questions 132–138

A 27-year-old man who has torn his anterior cruciate ligament (ACL) while skiing is sent to the operating room for ACL replacement and reconstruction. The anesthesiologist selects halothane.

132. Important adverse effects of halothane include all of the following EXCEPT

(A) depression of respiratory drive
(B) lowering of ventilatory response to carbon dioxide
(C) malignant hyperthermia in genetically sensitive individuals
(D) lowering of the seizure threshold
(E) depressed myocardial contractility

133. Induction of anesthesia is smooth, and the operation begins. Before any incision is made, the surgical resident informs the surgeon that this surgery is to be performed on the

(A) ankle
(B) knee
(C) hip
(D) elbow
(E) shoulder

134. The ACL stabilizes this joint by attaching the

(A) medial malleolus of the tibia to the talus
(B) lateral malleolus of the fibula to the talus
(C) head of the femur to the innominate (hip) bone
(D) femur to the fibula
(E) femur to the tibia

135. The head of the femur is attached to the innominate bone at the cup-shaped region known as the

(A) ilioischial fossa
(B) iliofemoral fossa
(C) ischial depression
(D) acetabulum
(E) sella turcica

136. The primary site of long bone growth occurs at the

(A) epiphysis
(B) diaphysis
(C) epiphyseal plate
(D) medullary cavity
(E) primary ossification center

137. All of the following bones are carpal bones EXCEPT

(A) capitate
(B) cuboid
(C) navicular
(D) trapezium
(E) trapezoid

138. All of the following statements are true for compact bone EXCEPT that it

(A) is made up of parallel bony columns
(B) contains neurovascular channels
(C) is composed of a network of trabeculae
(D) contains haversian canals
(E) contains osteocytes that communicate via gap junctions

139. Which of the following tests is contraindicated in patients with intracranial neoplasms?

(A) Computed tomography (CT) of the head because of the use of contrast dye
(B) Nuclear magnetic resonance (NMR) because of the length of time a patient must remain supine during testing
(C) Lumbar puncture to examine cerebrospinal proteins and relieve hydrocephalus
(D) X-ray imaging of the skull because the radiation may shrink the tumor and cause hemorrhaging

140. For the past 8 weeks, a scientist has developed rhinorrhea, conjunctival itching, a cough, and wheezing within 5–10 minutes of entering the animal facility where her experimental mice are housed. In the past week, she has begun to have wheezing and shortness of breath at night from 4–8 hours after working in the animal facility. Which of the following describes the late symptom complex? It is

(A) induced by mast cells triggered by rodent antigen with immunoglobulin E (IgE)
(B) a result of complement-mediated cytotoxicity
(C) not blocked by corticosteroids
(D) blocked by antihistamines

141. The figure below is a stylized diagram of the juxtaglomerular apparatus of the kidney. A decrease in the flow of glomerular filtrate into the tubules might cause which one of the following actions?

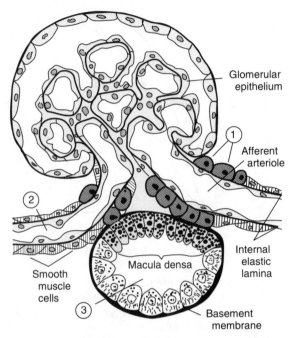

Glomerular epithelium

1 — Afferent arteriole

2

Internal elastic lamina

Macula densa

Smooth muscle cells

3

Basement membrane

(A) Renin released from *1*
(B) Vasodilation of *2*
(C) An increase in Na$^+$ concentration at *3*
(D) A reflexive vasoconstriction of the afferent arteriole

142. A quantitative Gram stain revealed many fewer cells than expected from the turbidity of a bacterial culture. The decrease in cells was most likely due to

(A) inactivation of the cytochromes
(B) digestion of the bacterial cell wall by autolytic processes
(C) presence of gram-negative organisms in the culture
(D) presence of bacterial spores in the culture

143. According to Fick's law, oxygen consumption is equal to the product of blood flow and arteriovenous oxygen difference. If the lungs absorb 300 ml/min of oxygen, arterial oxygen content is 20 ml/100 ml blood, pulmonary arterial oxygen content is 15 ml/100 ml blood, and heart rate is 60/min, then stroke volume is

(A) 50 ml
(B) 60 ml
(C) 100 ml
(D) 5 L/min
(E) 6 L/min

144. Capsule production is essential for the virulence of many pathogenic bacteria. Which of the following statements best describes bacterial capsules?

(A) The most important function of the *Streptococcus pneumoniae* capsule is adhesion
(B) The capsule of *Hemophilus influenzae* type B stimulates a T-cell–dependent immune response
(C) Opsonizing antibodies are often directed against *S. pneumoniae* capsules
(D) The capsule of group B *Neisseria meningitidis* is protein
(E) The DTP (diphtheria-tetanus-pertussis) vaccine currently licensed contains purified *Bordetella pertussis* capsules

145. True statements about the side chains of amino acids that are found in proteins include which one of the following?

(A) Serine provides strong buffering capacity at pH 7.0
(B) Alanine absorbs ultraviolet light
(C) Glutamic acid and aspartic acid differ significantly in their isoelectric pH (pI)
(D) Proline often produces a bend in the protein chain
(E) Only D-amino acids are incorporated into protein

146. Exogenous administration of large amounts of testosterone is likely to produce all of the following effects EXCEPT

(A) masculinization in mature females
(B) feminization in mature males
(C) closure of the epiphysis of long bones
(D) an increase in sperm count

147. A 56-year-old woman with a history of ovarian cancer treated by chemotherapy several years ago presents to a clinic with complaints of fatigue and the recent development of small hemorrhages on her arms. She has the following lab values: hemoglobin, 9.6 g/dl; white blood cells, 2900/μl; platelets, 56,000/μl. A bone marrow aspirate is hypercellular and contains approximately 10% blasts (normal < 5%) with megaloblastic morphologic changes in the red cell precursors and megakaryocytes with abnormal nuclei. Cytogenetic analysis reveals a clone with a deletion of the long arm of chromosome 7. What diagnosis best fits this woman's condition?

(A) Preleukemia (myelodysplastic syndrome)

(B) Megaloblastic anemia

(C) Acute lymphocytic leukemia

(D) Acute nonlymphocytic (myeloid) leukemia

(E) Chronic myelogenous leukemia

148. All of the following statements about collagen formation are true EXCEPT

(A) hydroxylation of proline requires molecular oxygen and α-ketoglutarate

(B) the triple helix forms after removal of the globular ends

(C) glycosylation occurs prior to hydroxylation

(D) assembly of tropocollagen into collagen fibrils is necessary for secretion

(E) the stability of the triple helix decreases with increasing hydroxyproline content

149. Of the drugs listed below, which one is thought to function through a receptor?

(A) Mannitol

(B) Dimercaprol

(C) Cimetidine

(D) Ethylenediaminetetraacetic acid (EDTA)

150. According to the figure below, which one of the following conditions would result in a shift of the oxygen saturation curve from *a* to *b*?

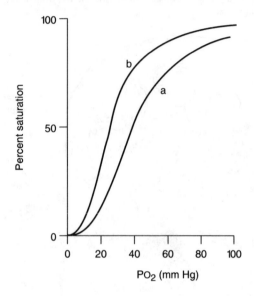

(A) A change in pH from 7.6 to 7.4

(B) A change in P_{CO_2} from 30 to 40 torr

(C) An increase in the concentration of 2,3-diphosphoglycerate (DPG)

(D) The presence of fetal hemoglobin ($\alpha_2\gamma_2$)

(E) The oxidation of the heme iron from Fe^{2+} to Fe^{3+}

151. All of the following statements about RNA are correct EXCEPT

(A) a messenger RNA (mRNA) molecule is translated once and is then degraded
(B) ribosomal RNA (rRNA) is formed by transcription of a family of repeated nuclear genes
(C) the ribosome, which is a complex of RNA and protein, is the site of protein synthesis
(D) three different RNA polymerase enzymes are required for sustained protein synthesis in human cells
(E) transfer RNA (tRNA) molecules contain an anticodon loop that pairs with the triplet codon of mRNA

152. Which one of the following muscles raises the soft palate during swallowing?

(A) Levator veli palatini
(B) Palatoglossus
(C) Palatopharyngeus
(D) Superior constrictor

153. A 32-year-old man with a 10-year history of undifferentiated schizophrenia is observed pacing around the house and fidgeting whenever seated. Recently, he received his monthly injection of fluphenazine. He is unemployed and lives in a personal care boarding home. The most likely cause of his agitation is

(A) anxiety
(B) restless legs syndrome
(C) akathisia
(D) undiagnosed hyperthyroidism
(E) worsening psychosis

154. Which one of the following statements best describes chondroblasts?

(A) They are endosteal cells capable of secreting proteoglycan
(B) They are perichondrial cells capable of secreting type II collagen
(C) They are periosteal cells capable of secreting type I collagen
(D) They show little mitotic activity
(E) They are filled with rough endoplasmic reticulum but lack a Golgi apparatus

155. A previously healthy 27-year-old woman is seen because of a petechial rash. She denies any recent bleeding and has had no recent illnesses. Hemoglobin, hematocrit, and white blood cell counts are normal. Examination of the peripheral blood smear reveals normal red and white blood cells and is remarkable only for a paucity of platelets. The most likely diagnosis in this patient is

(A) aleukemic leukemia
(B) idiopathic thrombocytopenic purpura (ITP)
(C) Glanzmann's thrombasthenia
(D) amegakaryocytic thrombocytopenia
(E) drug-induced thrombocytopenia

Questions 156–161

A 50-year-old man presents to the emergency room with severe epigastric pain, low-grade fever, tachycardia, and mild hypotension. The patient relates a history of moderate to heavy social drinking. The chief resident suspects acute pancreatitis.

156. The single most important laboratory finding to confirm the diagnosis of pancreatitis would be

(A) hyperlipidemia
(B) hyperbilirubinemia
(C) elevated serum amylase
(D) elevated serum phospholipase A
(E) elevated serum alkaline phosphatase

157. Which of the following polypeptide hormones is stimulated by increased acid from the stomach and subsequently stimulates the release of pancreatic juice rich in electrolytes and water?

(A) Gastrin
(B) Secretin
(C) Cholecystokinin
(D) Pancreozymin
(E) Vasoactive intestinal polypeptide (VIP)

158. Which of the following hormones is produced by the duodenal and upper jejunal mucosa and stimulates the release of pancreatic juice rich in digestive enzymes?

(A) Cholecystokinin
(B) Secretin
(C) Glucagon
(D) Pancreatic polypeptide
(E) VIP

159. Neuronal control of pancreatic exocrine function is mediated by

(A) VIP
(B) dopamine
(C) serotonin
(D) substance P
(E) acetylcholine (ACh)

160. Of the following statements about secretin, a polypeptide that has a significant effect on pancreatic secretion, which one is correct?

(A) It is synthesized in the pancreatic acinar cells
(B) It causes the pancreas to secrete large amounts of enzyme
(C) Its release is caused by the presence of fats and amino acids in the upper small intestine
(D) It causes the pancreas to secrete large amounts of bicarbonate ion (HCO_3^-)
(E) It is stored in an active form within S cells of the duodenum

161. The principal reason that the pancreas does not autodigest is that

(A) proteolytic enzymes are secreted as proenzymes
(B) pancreatic acini and ducts secrete a protective mucopolysaccharide, which lines their walls
(C) the pancreas maintains a slightly alkaline pH, rendering the digestive enzymes inactive
(D) pancreatic parenchyma is high in hydroxyproline, which is resistant to proteolysis
(E) proper enzyme substrates are not present

162. A complement fixation test is performed on a patient's serum by first adding influenza type A virus antigen and then adding complement, followed by antibody-coated sheep red blood cells (SRBC), which are then lysed. A possible explanation for this would be

(A) the patient has no immunoglobulin E (IgE) or IgA anti-influenza type A antibodies
(B) the patient's serum possesses an antibody that cross-reacts with SRBC
(C) the patient has no complement fixable anti-influenza type A antibodies
(D) the patient's serum possesses high levels of IgM, which cause SRBC lysis

163. Volume and pressure (alveolar; pleural) for a normal respiratory cycle are shown in the figure below. Which one of the following statements about respiration is correct?

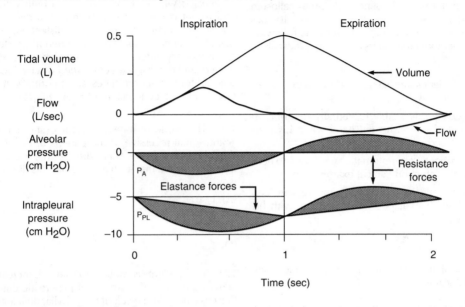

(A) Inspiration is the result of a passive process
(B) Gas flow is greatest at the end of inspiration
(C) Elastic recoil of the lung is identical at the beginning and end of inspiration
(D) During expiration, alveolar pressure becomes greater than atmospheric pressure

164. All of the following statements about hormone receptors are true EXCEPT that they

(A) may elicit their biologic response without being fully saturated with hormone
(B) may be desensitized by phosphorylation
(C) determine the specificity of cellular responses to hormones
(D) are deficient in Addison's disease
(E) are frequently transmembrane proteins

165. Which one of the following areas in a eukaryotic cell is a site of RNA processing?

(A) Mitochondria
(B) Golgi complex
(C) Rough endoplasmic reticulum
(D) Nuclear membrane

166. In humans, the major route of nitrogen metabolism from amino acids to urea involves which one of the following sets of enzymes?

(A) Amino acid oxidases and arginase
(B) Glutaminase and amino acid oxidases
(C) Glutamate dehydrogenase and transaminases
(D) Transaminases and glutaminase
(E) Glutamine synthetase and urease

167. A random subject undergoes magnetic resonance imaging (MRI) for an experiment, and a congenital malformation is found: The corpus callosum never developed, leaving the right and left sides of the brain unconnected. Which of the following statements about this man's condition is most likely to be true?

(A) The patient's intelligence and behavior are abnormal

(B) The patient is unable to verbally describe an object placed in his left hand when his eyes are closed

(C) The patient is asymptomatic and shows no neurologic defect on clinical examination

(D) The patient has a positive Romberg sign (i.e., he loses his balance when standing with his eyes closed)

168. All of the following statements concerning the subthalamus are true EXCEPT

(A) it contains the cranial ends of the nerve cells of the red nucleus

(B) it has important connections with the corpus striatum and, thus, is involved with voluntary muscle control

(C) it contains the cranial ends of the nerve cells of the substantia nigra

(D) it has important connections with the cerebellum and, thus, is involved with voluntary muscle control

169. Topoisomerase enzymes are important in the replication of DNA because they

(A) anneal Okazaki fragments

(B) relax supercoiled DNA

(C) degrade histone proteins

(D) "proofread" newly synthesized DNA

(E) synthesize the RNA primer fragment

Questions 170–172

A teenager who is below average in both weight and height is seen for complaints of vomiting of bile-stained material, abdominal distention, and pain. Further questioning reveals a periodic history of respiratory infections. Cystic fibrosis is suspected, and the diagnosis confirmed when pilocarpine iontophoresis produces an abnormally high sweat chloride concentration (> 60 mEq/L).

170. The mode of inheritance for cystic fibrosis is autosomal recessive. If the parents of the child described above are both disease-free carriers, then the chance that a sibling also has this disorder is

(A) 1/4

(B) 2/4

(C) 3/4

(D) 4/4

171. The patient is noted to have pancreatic achylia (absence of secretion of pancreatic digestive enzymes). As a result of the achylia, deficiency in absorption of which of the following vitamins may result in prolonged prothrombin times?

(A) Vitamin A

(B) Vitamin B_6

(C) Vitamin C

(D) Vitamin D

(E) Vitamin K

172. A history of frequent respiratory infections is noted in the patient. A recent sputum analysis indicates the presence of *Staphylococcus aureus, Hemophilus influenzae,* and *Pseudomonas aeruginosa.* Although the value of antibiotic therapy in cystic fibrosis remains unclear, a conventional approach to such therapy based on sputum culture might include

(A) gentamicin and ceftazidime

(B) nalidixic acid and kanamycin

(C) nitrofurantoin

(D) pentamidine

(E) rifampin and isoniazid

173. The micrograph below is of a portion of the liver biopsied from a 42-year-old man. The microscopic features seen are most likely due to

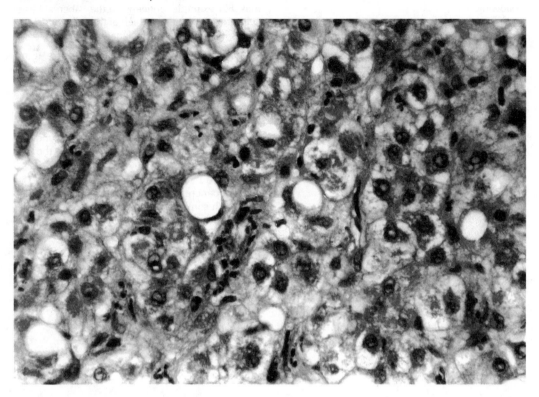

(A) exposure to carbon tetrachloride
(B) acetaminophen toxicity
(C) ethanol use
(D) acute rejection of a liver allograft

174. In the United States, the most common tumor in males is found in which one of the following organs?

(A) Kidney
(B) Colon
(C) Prostate gland
(D) Liver
(E) Testis

Questions 175–176

A patient is noted to have paroxysmal episodes of hypertension, tremor, weakness, and sweating. Urinary catecholamines and their metabolites are elevated, and a computed tomography (CT) scan of the abdomen detects a mass within the adrenal gland.

175. The tumor most likely involves which one of the following cells?

(A) Zona glomerulosa
(B) Zona fasciculata
(C) Zona reticularis
(D) Chromaffin cells of the medulla

176. If the tumor is deemed inoperable, pharmacotherapy of the above disorder may include which one of the following drugs?

(A) Clonidine
(B) Propranolol
(C) Methyldopa
(D) Phenoxybenzamine

177. Correct statements concerning toxic exposure to organophosphates include which one of the following?

(A) Aminophylline is the agent of first choice in reversing the respiratory symptoms

(B) Atropine and pralidoxime are useful antidotes

(C) Exposure must be inhalational since organophosphates are not well absorbed through the skin

(D) Immediate injection of epinephrine is a useful antidote

178. In general, tolerance to self-antigens exists, even if the antigens are not expressed in the thymus. For example, antigens on the pancreatic islet cells produce insulin. Which of the following statements is a reasonable explanation for this?

(A) Pancreatic antigens are shed and are transported to the thymus via the circulation; at the thymus, they are associated with the major histocompatability complex (MHC) and induce positive selection of immature T cells

(B) Immature CD4$^+$CD8$^+$ thymic T cells are transported to the pancreas, where they undergo negative selection; they then return to the thymus for final maturation

(C) Mature T cells circulate to the pancreas, recognize pancreatic antigen in context of self MHC, which stimulates them via the T-cell receptor; however, no interleukin-1 is produced, so T cells are inactivated

(D) T-cell progenitors in the bone marrow circulate to the pancreas before being transported to the thymus; they undergo negative selection at the pancreas and then proceed to the thymus where T-cell differentiation occurs

Directions: Each group of items in this section consists of lettered options followed by a set of numbered items. For each item, select the **one** lettered option that is most closely associated with it. Each lettered option may be selected once, more than once, or not at all.

Questions 179–183

Match each of the following structures with its germ layer of origin.

(A) Ectoderm
(B) Mesoderm
(C) Endoderm
(D) Neuroectoderm

179. Melanocytes

180. Adrenal cortex

181. Liver

182. Thyroid gland

183. Gonads

Questions 184–186

Match each description below with the appropriate lettered structure in the scanning electron micrograph of liver parenchymal tissue.

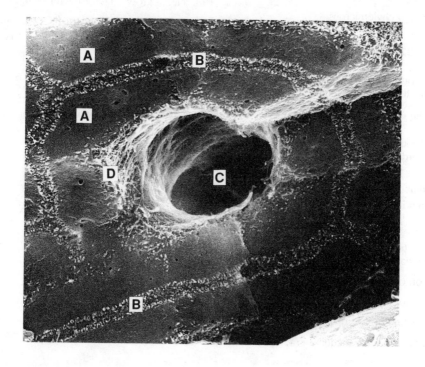

184. Receives blood from the portal vein and hepatic artery and drains blood into the central vein

185. A liver parenchymal cell

186. A bile canaliculus surrounded by tight junctions that form the blood–bile barrier

Questions 187–191

For each lipoprotein type listed below, select the genetic disorder that is most likely to be associated with it.

(A) Combined hyperlipidemia
(B) Hypertriglyceridemia
(C) Type III hyperlipoproteinemia
(D) Hypercholesterolemia
(E) Lipoprotein lipase deficiency

187. Chylomicrons

188. Low-density lipoproteins (LDL)

189. Chylomicron remnants and intermediate-density lipoproteins (IDL)

190. Very low-density lipoproteins (VLDL)

191. VLDL and chylomicrons

Questions 192–196

Match each procedure or operation with the neurotransmitter that it would deplete.

(A) Serotonin and catecholamines in the cerebral cortex
(B) γ-Aminobutyric acid (GABA) and glycine in the spinal cord
(C) Substance P in the dorsal horns
(D) Dopamine in the basal ganglia
(E) Serotonin in the spinal cord

192. Destruction of spinal interneurons (by controlled hypoxia)

193. Section of dorsal roots

194. Section of the medial forebrain bundle

195. Destruction of the substantia nigra

196. Destruction of the medullary raphe

Questions 197–200

Oncogenesis, the production of tumors, occurs due to the loss of cellular signaling, which is frequently caused by a protein that functions as an uncontrolled growth factor receptor. Match the normal physiologic receptor with the oncogene that it most closely resembles functionally and structurally.

(A) *ros*
(B) *erbB*
(C) *trk*
(D) *sis*
(E) *kit*
(F) *jun*

197. Insulin receptor

198. Nerve growth factor (NGF) receptor

199. Epidermal growth factor (EGF) receptor

200. Platelet-derived growth factor (PDGF) receptor

Questions 201–206

Match each disease below with its etiologic agent.

(A) *Treponema pallidum*
(B) *Treponema pertenue*
(C) *Treponema carateum*
(D) *Leptospira interrogans*
(E) *Borrelia recurrentis*

201. Relapsing fever

202. Bejel

203. Pinta

204. Syphilis

205. Fort Bragg fever

206. Yaws

Questions 207–212

The first heart sound (S_1) is composed of sounds from tricuspid and mitral valve closure. The second heart sound (S_2) is the sound of the aortic and pulmonic valves closing. For each cardiovascular abnormality listed below, select the heart sounds with which it is most likely to be associated.

(A) S_1 louder than S_2
(B) S_2 louder than S_1
(C) Aortic valvular ejection sound
(D) Pulmonic valvular ejection sound

207. Mitral valve stenosis

208. Aortic stenosis

209. Acute aortic regurgitation

210. Severe hypertension

211. Anemia

212. Hyperthyroidism

Questions 213–216

Match the forms of joint disease listed below with the characteristic typically associated with it.

(A) Onion-skin thickening of the arterioles
(B) Tophus
(C) Human leukocyte antigen DR4 (HLA-DR4)
(D) Heberden's nodes

213. Rheumatoid arthritis

214. Osteoarthritis

215. Lyme arthritis

216. Gouty arthritis

Questions 217–219

The esophageal and arterial pressure tracings below were made from a normal subject during a voluntary effort to exhale against significant resistance (the Valsalva maneuver), which is a useful test of cardiac function. Match the descriptions that follow with the labeled arterial pressure readings.

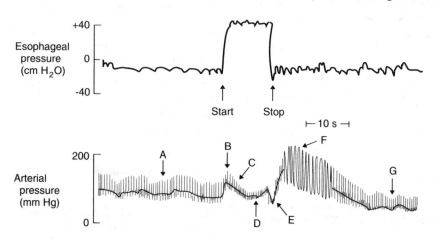

217. Loss of this vagally mediated change in arterial pressure is a useful diagnostic aid in assessing autonomic insufficiency

218. Changes in arterial blood pressure and pulse pressure are due to a decrease in venous return

219. This area of the arterial blood pressure tracing is consistent with reflex tachycardia

Questions 220–224

Match each disease characteristic with the personality disorder that is most apt to be associated with it.

(A) Obsessive–compulsive
(B) Borderline
(C) Dependent
(D) Narcissistic
(E) Antisocial

220. Associated with childhood conduct disorder

221. Overly rigid

222. Hypersensitive to criticism

223. Repetitive self-cutting

224. Perfectionistic

Questions 225–227

Match each phrase describing a feature of inflammatory heart disease with the disease it characterizes.

(A) Acute rheumatic fever
(B) Chronic rheumatic heart disease
(C) Acute bacterial endocarditis
(D) Subacute bacterial endocarditis
(E) Libman-Sacks endocarditis

225. Fusion of the commissures

226. Infection by group A β-hemolytic streptococci

227. Infection by α-hemolytic (viridans) streptococci

Questions 228–232

Based on the clinical information given, select the bone tumor that is most likely to occur in each patient.

(A) Osteosarcoma
(B) Chondrosarcoma
(C) Ewing's sarcoma
(D) Giant cell tumor
(E) Osteoid osteoma
(F) Chondroblastoma

228. Epiphyseal lesions in a patient less than 20 years old

229. Epiphyseal lesions in a patient more than 20 years old

230. Metaphyseal lesions in a patient less than 20 years old

231. A radiolucent nidus surrounded by sclerotic bone in a patient less than 20 years old

232. A diaphyseal lesion with concentric onion-skin layering in a patient less than 20 years old

Questions 233–235

Match each description below with the most appropriate abdominal fascia.

(A) Camper's fascia
(B) Scarpa's fascia
(C) Both
(D) Neither

233. Prominent over the abdominal wall

234. Supports sutures

235. Called Colles' fascia in the perineum

Questions 236–243

Match each pathologic feature listed below with the idiopathic inflammatory bowel disease of which it is most characteristic.

(A) Ulcerative colitis
(B) Crohn's disease
(C) Whipple's disease
(D) Hirschsprung's disease

236. Segmental lesions

237. Fistulae

238. Periodic acid–Schiff (PAS)-positive macrophages in the lamina propria

239. Megacolon

240. Crypt abscesses

241. Granulomas

242. Superficial ulceration

243. Transmural inflammation

Questions 244–247

For each characteristic of lung carcinoma listed below, select the corresponding tumor.

(A) Adenocarcinoma
(B) Squamous cell carcinoma
(C) Small cell carcinoma
(D) Bronchioloalveolar adenocarcinoma

244. Associated with the *ras* oncogene amplification and mutation

245. Presence of neurosecretory granules

246. Similar to jaagsiekte disease in sheep

247. Association with the *myc* oncogene amplification and mutation

Questions 248–252

Match each of the following diseases that affect the brain with its most characteristic neuropathologic finding.

(A) Lewy bodies
(B) Hippocampal neurofibrillary tangles
(C) Argentophilic intraneuronal inclusions
(D) Prions
(E) Multinucleated giant cells

248. Alzheimer's dementia

249. AIDS

250. Parkinson's disease

251. Creutzfeldt-Jakob disease

252. Pick's disease

Questions 253–257

Match each of the following descriptions of neurochemistry with the enzyme that is most likely to be associated with it.

(A) Tyrosine hydroxylase
(B) Monoamine oxidase (MAO)
(C) Choline acetyltransferase
(D) Tryptophan-5-hydroxylase
(E) Catechol-O-methyltransferase

253. Decreased in Alzheimer's dementia

254. Rate-limiting step for catecholamine synthesis

255. Located on the mitochondrial membrane

256. Levels increase with increasing age

257. Found in neurons of the dorsal raphe nuclei

ANSWER KEY

1-E	31-D	61-E	91-A	121-C
2-E	32-D	62-A	92-C	122-D
3-C	33-A	63-C	93-E	123-B
4-D	34-D	64-E	94-D	124-E
5-A	35-D	65-B	95-C	125-C
6-B	36-A	66-B	96-C	126-A
7-E	37-A	67-B	97-D	127-E
8-A	38-A	68-D	98-C	128-B
9-C	39-E	69-E	99-A	129-D
10-A	40-D	70-D	100-C	130-A
11-D	41-C	71-D	101-E	131-C
12-C	42-C	72-A	102-A	132-D
13-B	43-C	73-C	103-B	133-B
14-C	44-D	74-E	104-C	134-E
15-B	45-C	75-C	105-B	135-D
16-D	46-E	76-E	106-C	136-C
17-A	47-E	77-E	107-B	137-B
18-C	48-A	78-B	108-B	138-C
19-A	49-D	79-C	109-B	139-C
20-D	50-B	80-C	110-E	140-A
21-B	51-C	81-C	111-B	141-A
22-B	52-A	82-C	112-D	142-D
23-B	53-D	83-C	113-A	143-C
24-C	54-D	84-C	114-C	144-C
25-A	55-D	85-D	115-C	145-D
26-D	56-B	86-B	116-B	146-D
27-B	57-E	87-C	117-A	147-A
28-E	58-B	88-B	118-C	148-D
29-D	59-C	89-E	119-D	149-C
30-A	60-D	90-D	120-D	150-D

151-A	173-C	195-D	216-B	237-B
152-A	174-C	196-E	217-F	238-C
153-C	175-D	197-A	218-C	239-D
154-B	176-D	198-C	219-D	240-A
155-B	177-B	199-B	220-E	241-B
156-C	178-C	200-E	221-A	242-A
157-B	179-D	201-E	222-D	243-B
158-A	180-B	202-A	223-B	244-A
159-E	181-C	203-C	224-A	245-C
160-D	182-C	204-A	225-B	246-D
161-A	183-B	205-D	226-A	247-C
162-C	184-C	206-B	227-D	248-B
163-D	185-A	207-A	228-F	249-E
164-D	186-B	208-C	229-D	250-A
165-A	187-E	209-B	230-A	251-D
166-C	188-D	210-B	231-E	252-C
167-C	189-C	211-A	232-C	253-C
168-D	190-B	212-A	233-C	254-A
169-B	191-A	213-C	234-B	255-B
170-A	192-B	214-D	235-B	256-B
171-E	193-C	215-A	236-B	257-D
172-A	194-A			

ANSWERS AND EXPLANATIONS

1. The answer is E. *(Protein structure; receptors)*
Known receptors for physiologic growth factors and effectors display a small group of structures that are shared among different proteins and are found on either the external or internal domain of the protein. These structures are recognizable at a primary amino acid sequence level. This allows receptors to be classified into groups that resemble ion channels; groups that resemble kinases, especially tyrosine, serine, and threonine kinases; and cyclases. Several plasma membrane receptors require interactions with guanosine triphosphate (GTP)–binding proteins (G proteins) to function in signal transduction. Metallothionin is a good acceptor for zinc and heavy metal, but it has not been reported to be a receptor or an element in signal transduction systems.

2. The answer is E. *(Neurotransmitters; excitatory amino acids)*
Decreased GABA-ergic activity is associated with increased seizure activity, and antiepileptic drugs are GABA-ergic. Baclofen, used for multiple sclerosis, reduces muscle spasms. Benzodiazepines have agonist activity at a macromolecular receptor complex that includes a γ-aminobutyric acid (GABA) receptor, and the activity of this receptor appears to be overactive in hepatic encephalopathy.

3–7. The answers are: 3-C, 4-D, 5-A, 6-B, 7-E. *(Duchenne muscular dystrophy)*
Duchenne muscular dystrophy (DMD), or childhood muscular dystrophy, classically occurs only in boys with a pattern of X-linked inheritance. This pattern can be deduced from the pedigree that accompanies the question because all of the affected individuals are males, the mothers and fathers are not affected, and the affected males are on the maternal side of the family.

In X-linked diseases, mothers are always carriers because the mutant gene is on the X chromosome. The male child either receives the X chromosome with the mutant gene and gets the disease or receives a normal X chromosome and does not get the disease. Males cannot be carriers of X-linked disorders. A female carrier has a 50% chance of giving her chromosome that bears the mutant gene to each of her children.

The gene mutation that causes DMD occurs in the dystrophin gene, which is a very large gene located on the short arm of the X chromosome. Most mutations involve deletions of varying lengths. Dystrophin is similar to the cytoskeletal proteins actin and spectrin, both of which are normal in this disease. It is thought that dystrophin plays a role in controlling calcium release, but its true function has not yet been elucidated.

The diagnosis of DMD is confirmed by electromyography, measurement of creatine kinase (CK), which is increased tenfold, and muscle biopsy. CK levels can be measured at birth if DMD is suspected on the basis of family history, but intrauterine diagnosis of all cases of DMD is not yet possible because of the number and types of mutations that occur.

8. The answer is A. *(Hypocomplementemia-associated renal disease)*
Complement levels are normal in immunoglobulin A (IgA) nephropathy and diffuse proliferative glomerulonephritis (poststreptococcal glomerulonephritis). Nephrides associated with hypocomplementemia include cryoglobulinemia, membranoproliferative glomerulonephropathy, and a variety of visceral infections, including infections of peritoneal and central nervous system (CNS) shunts ("shunt" nephritis).

9. The answer is C. *(Histopathology of Kaposi's sarcoma)*
Kaposi's sarcoma was initially described as a cutaneous hemorrhagic nodule usually occurring on the lower extremities of elderly men. With the AIDS epidemic, Kaposi's sarcoma is now recognized as being associated with human immunodeficiency virus (HIV) infection and afflicting many homosexual men. It is recognized histologically by irregular fascicles of spindle cells in the dermis, which are accompanied by extravasated erythrocytes that impart a purple color. Kaposi's sarcoma is believed to be derived from endothelial cells, perhaps lymphatic endothelium. Unlike angiosarcomas, it does not form anastomosing vascular channels.

10. The answer is A. *(Referred pain)*
Referred pain is not well understood. Somatic referred pain is very well localized and intense. Visceral referred pain is the opposite and is thought to be conveyed by autonomic fibers. Diaphragmatic pain is usually referred to the shoulder.

11–13. The answers are: 11-D, 12-C, 13-B. *(Diagnosis and pharmacology of epilepsy)*
Major depression is the first diagnosis to consider because, in the case presented in the question, the subacute time course, self-neglect, social withdrawal, and psychotic symptoms indicate a possible

depression. Major depression, even depression associated with psychotic symptoms, is treatable and has a good prognosis. There is no mention of drug abuse to suggest phencyclidine psychosis and no euphoria or increased sociability to suggest mania. The time during which symptoms have occurred has not been long enough to suggest schizophrenia or schizoaffective disorder.

The symptoms listed in the questions suggest complex partial seizures of the temporal lobe. Considering the psychotic symptoms and social withdrawal, epilepsy with schizophreniform interictal disorder might also be considered. The evoked potentials and the projective or cognitive tests would not be helpful.

Carbamazepine is the preferred treatment for complex partial seizures. The antipsychotic drug haloperidol should be added only if the psychotic symptoms do not respond to the antiepileptic agent. Haloperidol and the antidepressant imipramine lower the seizure threshold. The antipanic drug alprazolam is not indicated, although some other types of benzodiazepines are used as antiepileptics.

14. The answer is C. *(Inflammation and cellular margination)*
As the vascular phase of the inflammatory response progresses, neutrophils and monocytes move toward the periphery of the microcirculatory vessels (a process referred to as margination) and then adhere to, or pavement, the vascular endothelium in preparation for migration into the extravascular space. To migrate, leukocytes develop pseudopods and move, without accompanying loss of fluid, through gaps between the endothelial cells — a process termed diapedesis. In the latter part of the vascular phase, increased vascular permeability causes loss of plasma with resultant venous stasis and, eventually, clotting in the small capillaries local to the inflamed area.

15. The answer is B. *(Hormone receptors)*
The cytosol would contain the most fluorescence. Glucocorticoid receptors are soluble receptors and are not associated with the plasma membrane. Glucocorticoids diffuse into cells, bind to receptors in the cytosol, and then translocate to the nucleus. Inside the nucleus this hormone-receptor complex regulates transcription via binding to specific sequences of DNA.

16. The answer is D. *(Immunologic disorders)*
The major histocompatibility complex, which is also known as the human leukocyte antigen (HLA) complex, has been associated with a variety of diseases. Probably the best known association is between HLA-B27 and ankylosing spondylitis. All of the HLA associations in the question are matched correctly except for 21-hydroxylase deficiency, which is associated with HLA-BW47, not HLA-DR4.

17. The answer is A. *(Histopathology of temporal arteritis)*
Temporal (giant cell) arteritis may be one component of the syndrome of polymyalgia rheumatica. Patients present with headache, tenderness over the temporal artery, visual loss (if retinal vessels are affected), and facial pain. Histologically, a granulomatous reaction is seen within the vessel wall associated with a mixed neutrophilic and lymphocytic infiltrate. Giant cells appear to phagocytize portions of elastica, and the vessel may be thrombosed in its late stage *(right)*. Clinical response to steroids is excellent. Mönckeberg's arteriosclerosis shows medial calcification of arteries and is not an arteritis, while Takayasu's arteritis ("pulseless disease") involves the aortic arch and its major branches.

18. The answer is C. *(Asthma and pharmacology of cromolyn sodium)*
Cromolyn sodium inhibits degranulation of mast cells and, in other poorly understood ways, interferes with the inflammatory process now assumed to be critical to moderate asthma due to a variety of allergens and other conditions. Cromolyn is not absorbed from the gut and must be administered topically to the lung where it acts prophylactically to inhibit bronchospasm due to inhaled allergens, exercise, or altered environmental conditions. It does not directly relax bronchial smooth muscle in vivo or in vitro and, thus, is of little use in acute emergencies of bronchial hyperreactivity. However, prophylactically, it will reduce the bronchial response to a number of spasmogens.

19–20. The answers are: 19-A, 20-D. *(Diagnosis and pathology of acute leukemia)*
The presence of pancytopenia is not associated with chronic lymphocytic leukemia. Patients with acute myelogenous leukemia, recurrent ovarian carcinoma, and aplastic anemia can have pancytopenia. Cyclophosphamide, which is used to treat some patients with ovarian carcinoma, does cause bone marrow depression, and recovery can be delayed.

An immunoglobulin gene rearrangement analysis would not be useful for this patient unless she had shown evidence of a lymphoproliferative disorder. Radiographic and cytologic studies could confirm the presence of ascites and possible recurrent ovarian carcinoma. Bone marrow aspiration is essential to establish the diagnosis. With hepatic enlargement, it is necessary to evaluate the patient for evidence of liver damage. Some agents that damage the liver can also damage the bone marrow.

21. The answer is B. *(Asthma; pulmonary mechanics)*
The forced vital capacity (FVC) is unchanged or decreased during an acute asthma attack. An important spirometric manifestation of asthma is a decrease in forced expiratory volume in 1 second (FEV_1) by itself or normalized to FVC. Total lung capacity (TLC) will be normal, or elevated possibly, because of loss of elastic recoil.

22. The answer is B. *(Histology of liquefactive necrosis)*
Coagulative necrosis follows hypoxic death in most body tissues except those of the central nervous system (CNS). For example, the necrotic process that ensues following a myocardial infarction is coagulative necrosis, due to occlusion of the coronary vessels. Liquefactive necrosis occurs only in the CNS, as a result of vascular occlusion. It is more commonly caused by pyogenic bacterial infection or septic emboli.

23–26. The answers are: 23-B, 24-C, 25-A, 26-D. *(Gastric ulcer disease)*
A number of physiologic, genetic, and other factors increase the risk of gastric (and duodenal) peptic ulcers. Smoking and caffeine are known to adversely affect the morbidity, mortality, and healing rate of peptic ulcers. In general, first-degree relatives of peptic ulcer patients as well as males have a threefold to fourfold increased risk of developing this disorder. Paradoxically, in gastric ulcer disease, acid secretion is not elevated. It is possible that excess secreted hydrogen ion is reabsorbed across the injured gastric mucosa. In general, a defect in gastric mucosal defense is the more important local physiologic factor promoting ulceration at this site.

In the patient described in the question, direct visualization identified a duodenal ulcer, a very common cause of right upper quadrant pain and melena. Denudation of the mucosal epithelium is the hallmark of histologic changes in peptic ulcer disease and, in duodenal ulcer, is often accompanied by hypertrophy of submucosal Brunner's glands (mucus-secreting glands).

The agents of choice for duodenal ulcer include histamine (H_2) antagonists, including ranitidine or cimetidine. Other useful agents, alone or in combination with H_2 antagonists, include anticholinergic drugs, "proton pump" inhibitors (benzimidazoles), antacids, and cytoprotective analogues of prostaglandins E_1, E_2, and prostacyclin.

27. The answer is B. *(Tumor pathology)*
In most human cancers, the stage of the disease, not the age of the patient, is the most important prognostic factor. Stage refers to the extent, or degree of spread, of the disease in the patient (i.e., localized, regional, or distant). Tumor grade (i.e., differentiation), mitotic count, and extent of invasion correlate with the stage of the tumor, in that high-grade (i.e., less differentiated) tumors and highly invasive tumors tend to be high-stage lesions.

28. The answer is E. *(Telencephalon)*
Elements that develop from the telencephalon, which includes the internal capsule and the area lateral to it, include the forebrain; parietal, temporal, and occipital lobes; the hippocampus; and the corpus striatum. The thalamus is considered part of the diencephalon.

29. The answer is D. *(Growth hormone)*
Growth hormone stimulates cartilage and bone growth via somatomedin, an intermediary peptide. It is secreted periodically, like many other pituitary hormones, and is affected in a negative fashion by somatostatin, a hypothalamic peptide. Unlike other anterior pituitary hormones, cellular targets for growth hormone are relatively ubiquitous. Somatomedin, synthesized in the liver and possibly other sites (e.g., muscle), is an important mediator of the growth effects of the hormone on cartilage and bone. Indeed, growth hormone has no direct effects on these cells by itself. Growth hormone has a large array of effects on amino acid, fat, and carbohydrate activities and, in general, displays anti–insulin-like actions.

30. The answer is A. *(Skeletal muscle contraction)*
The length of the A band remains constant during the contraction of myofibrils in skeletal muscle. The sarcomere of the myofibril is composed of thick and thin filaments. According to the sliding filament hypothesis, thick and thin filaments slide past one another during contraction, increasing the amount of overlap between them; they do not change length. The H band contains only thick filaments; the A band contains thin and thick filaments. The I band contains only thin filaments, which are anchored in the middle of the I band by components of the Z disk. During contraction, thin filaments slide into the A band, reducing the size of both the H band and I band and drawing the Z disks closer to the A band.

31. The answer is D. *(Diagnosis of pneumocystis pneumonia)*
Pneumocystis pneumonia is caused by *Pneumocystis carinii*, a microorganism of uncertain classification that belongs to either the protozoa or fungi. It forms four to seven microcysts within a frothy honeycomb-like alveolar exudate in the air spaces. These cysts contain numerous sporozoites, which are released from the cysts at maturation. Pneumocystis pneumonia is commonly seen in individuals infected with human immunodeficiency virus (HIV), a condition that would be suspected in an individual with a history of intravenous drug abuse.

32. The answer is D. *(Histopathology of Hodgkin's disease)*
The photomicrograph of the woman's biopsy shows classic features of nodular-sclerosing Hodgkin's disease. The node is divided into irregular nodules by broad bands of dense collagen *(left)*. In the panel on the *right,* the nodal infiltrate is composed of lymphocytes, plasma cells, eosinophils, and multilobated cells with prominent red nucleoli called Reed-Sternberg cells. While Reed-Sternberg cells are not pathognomonic of this disease, they are diagnostic when seen in this appropriate inflammatory milieu. The nodular sclerosis type of Hodgkin's disease usually presents with a large mediastinal mass and involvement of adjacent lymph node groups (e.g., supraclavicular nodes).

33. The answer is A. *(Na$^+$ transport and renal epithelial physiology)*
Na$^+$ is transported from the tubular lumen to the peritubular capillary by an electrochemical gradient that is largely generated by the action of the Na$^+$, K$^+$-ATPase activity at the basolateral surface. The cell is freely permeable to water and chloride, thereby reabsorbing a virtually isosmotic fraction of tubular luminal fluid. The attraction of Na$^+$ creates a very large intracellular negative potential (approximately -70 mV). There is no significant hormone dependence of ion transport in these cells on either aldosterone or antidiuretic hormone (ADH).

34. The answer is D. *(Thoracic outlet syndrome)*
Thoracic outlet syndrome describes compression of the lower trunk of the brachial plexus and the subclavian artery by an anomalous thirteenth (cervical) rib. Sensory changes occur over the distribution of the ulnar nerve; the phrenic nerves are not involved.

35. The answer is D. *(Gluconeogenesis and glycolysis)*
Stimulation of beta cells by glucose results in the release of insulin. Insulin has numerous effects on virtually every tissue, and its overall effect is the conservation of body fuel supplies. It does this by promoting the uptake and storage of glucose, amino acids, and fats. In the liver, it decreases gluconeogenesis and glycogenolysis and promotes glycolysis. In addition, it promotes lipogenesis in the liver and fat cells and is antilipolytic. It is also an important anabolic protein hormone while simultaneously inhibiting the breakdown of amino acids. It inhibits the release of glucagon from neighboring alpha cells.

36. The answer is A. *(Intercostal nerves)*
Intercostal nerves are the anterior rami of the first 11 thoracic spinal nerves; the twelfth thoracic nerve gives rise to the subcostal nerve.

37. The answer is A. *(Cranial injury)*
The amount of injury to the brain is proportional to the amount of distance the brain moves within the skull before being forcibly halted by fixed structures within the skull. Blows to the front or back of the head cause more displacement of the brain and, hence, more trauma than blows directed to the side of the head. A blow that glances off the head causes considerable rotation of the brain within the skull and, thus, is potentially more dangerous than blows to the sides, front, or back of the head.

38–39. The answers are: 38-A, 39-E. *(Multiple myeloma; immunoglobulin abnormalities)*
Well-demarcated or "punched out" osteolytic lesions are almost pathognomonic for multiple myeloma. In 99% of the patients with multiple myeloma, electrophoretic analysis of the serum proteins shows an increase in one of the immunoglobulin classes or light chains, approximately 23,000 daltons (Bence Jones protein), in the urine. The presence of 55,000-dalton monoclonal proteins is indicative of heavy-chain disease, a different type of monoclonal gammapathy that is not associated with osteolytic lesions. Although not specific for this disease, patients with multiple myeloma do suffer from a suppression of synthesis of normal antibodies and are, thus, susceptible to recurrent bacterial and viral infections.

In approximately 55% of people diagnosed with multiple myeloma, the membrane-bound protein (M protein) is immunoglobulin G (IgG), and in 25%, the M protein is IgA and rarely IgM, IgD, or IgE. In the remaining 20%, Bence Jones proteinuria without the serum M protein is seen.

40. The answer is D. *(Pharmacology of aminoglycosides)*
Aminoglycosides can cause severe nephrotoxicity and ototoxicity. Their therapeutic index is low; peak and trough levels are commonly monitored to allow for dose adjustments or a change in timing of administration. Aminoglycosides are eliminated rapidly with a serum half-life of 1–5 hours. However, rapid clearance is not the major determinant for therapeutic monitoring. Aminoglycosides are not extensively metabolized. Since they are polar molecules, they are lipid insoluble and do not cross the blood–brain barrier. The incidence of hypersensitivity reactions is extremely low.

41. The answer is C. *(Neoplasia and hormone action)*
Tamoxifen has become the drug of choice for the initial endocrine management of breast cancer as well as a useful adjuvant therapy for the palliative management of advanced breast cancer. It is relatively nontoxic, and patients with breast tumors containing estrogen receptors are most likely to respond to the drug. The drug binds to the estrogen receptor in the nucleus but does not stimulate transcription. The tamoxifen–estrogen receptor complex does not readily dissociate, thereby affecting estrogen receptor recycling. In premenopausal women, competition with estrogen receptors in the anterior pituitary and hypothalamus disrupts normal feedback inhibition of gonadotropin-releasing hormone, thereby enhancing gonadotropin release.

42. The answer is C. *(Angina therapy)*
Nitroglycerin (glyceryl trinitrate; GTN) is most effective by decreasing preload in angina. At high concentrations, some benefit in angina is obtained from GTN by reducing afterload. However, this latter effect is often accompanied by reflex tachycardia that may disrupt the improvement in myocardial oxygen consumption and supply achieved by GTN. Propranolol is useful in blocking this reflex effect since it is negatively inotropic and negatively chronotropic. Propranolol may be accompanied by coronary artery vasospasm after removing β-receptor–mediated dilation and leaving unopposed a coronary artery α-receptor–mediated vasoconstriction.

43. The answer is C. *(Antiepileptics)*
Phenytoin decreases resting Na^+ flux as well as the flow of Na^+ currents during chemical depolarization or action potential. In the central nervous system (CNS), this results in depression of the generation and transmission of repetitive action potentials in epileptic foci. It is usually the drug of choice for all seizures except absence seizures and, in general, is started alone to assess its efficacy. Phenytoin is associated with potential teratogenic effects (fetal hydantoin syndrome). Other agents like diazepam or phenobarbital affect chloride channels by interacting with γ-aminobutyric acid (GABA) at its receptor site.

44. The answer is D. *(RNA synthesis)*
RNA polymerase I produces ribosomal RNA (rRNA). RNA polymerase II produces mostly messenger RNA (mRNA). RNA polymerase III makes transfer RNA (tRNA) and other small RNAs. The reason that mammalian cells use three different types of RNA polymerases is not known.

45. The answer is C. *(Toxicology and aplastic anemia)*
Benzene is associated with the induction of aplastic anemia by damaging myeloid stem cells. Thiouracil is associated with agranulocytosis, primarily due to its ability to decrease production or increase destruction of neutrophils. Penicillin acts as a hapten, which produces erythrocyte destruction via warm antibody autoimmune hemolysis. In contrast, methyldopa stimulates the production of antibodies against intrinsic red blood cell antigens. Ingestion of an excessive quantity of acetaminophen is followed by the production of toxic metabolites, which first decrease hepatic glutathione levels and then cause a centrilobular necrosis due to biomolecular adduct formation.

46. The answer is E. *(Monoclonal antibodies and gram-negative bacteria)*
A monoclonal antibody, such as immunoglobulin G (IgG), against endotoxin would be useful only against an organism producing lipopolysaccharide, namely gram-negative bacteria. The organism would have to produce a disease state through bacteremia since IgG would only be present in the circulatory system. Organisms such as *Bordetella pertussis*, the causative agent of whooping cough, and *Vibrio cholerae*, the agent of cholera, are gram-negative but do not invade the bloodstream. Pulmonary anthrax is caused by *Bacillus anthracis*, which is a gram-positive organism. Leprosy is caused by *Mycobacterium leprae*, which is acid-fast, not gram-negative. Bubonic plague, however, is caused by *Yersinia pestis*, a gram-negative organism that multiplies in the bloodstream, spreading through to the lymphatics. *Y. pestis* has many virulence factors, including lipopolysaccharide.

47. The answer is E. *(Mechanism of action of penicillin)*
The principles of antibiotic action are perhaps best exemplified by penicillin. Antibiotics act by specifically binding to macromolecules only found in the parasite. Transpeptidase is the only penicillin-binding protein listed; it is inactivated when binding occurs.

48. The answer is A. *(Transcriptional activation of chromosomes)*
Mammalian DNA utilizes only about 7% of the genome to transcribe RNA. Inactive DNA is referred to as heterochromatin, and it is tightly wound in an organized fashion in conjunction with nucleosomes. Inactive DNA is also methylated at CG islands, but the exact relation between inactivation and methylation is not clear. Active segments of DNA are referred to as euchromatin. Euchromatin is not wound as tightly and is less protein bound than heterochromatin. Because it is less organized, euchromatin also happens to be more sensitive to enzymatic digestion by DNase I, which can be used to determine active regions of DNA.

49. The answer is D. *(Passive immunity; vaccination)*
The most appropriate treatment for the medical student described in the question would be an injection of tetanus toxoid, which would trigger an anamnestic response because of the DTP (diphtheria-tetanus-pertussis) administration in childhood. If there is no history of DTP immunization, passive immunity can be induced by the administration of heterologous (e.g., equine) or homologous (i.e., human) antibodies. Type I and type III reactions can result from heterologous administration. Aminoglycosides are given for infections due to gram-negative bacteria. The tetanus toxoid is produced by *Clostridium tetani*, a gram-positive rod.

50. The answer is B. *(Adverse effects of aspirin)*
The major adverse effect of aspirin is gastrointestinal bleeding. Inhibition of local cytoprotective arachidonic acid metabolites (prostaglandin E_2 and prostacyclin) in the gastric mucosa contributes to this adverse effect and can be offset by simultaneously using exogenous synthetic prostanoids. In addition, aspirin has a direct irritating effect on the mucosa. Nonsteroidal anti-inflammatory agents in general have little effect on lipoxygenase activity but do affect cyclooxygenase. In particular, aspirin is an irreversible inhibitor of this enzyme in platelets (and other cell types) by acetylating the α-amino group of the terminal serine. This irreversible inhibition has significant implications in that platelet function will not be restored to normal until a new enzyme has been synthesized. Aspirin has little effect on normal body temperature but reduces abnormally elevated body temperatures secondary to alterations in central thermoregulation.

51. The answer is C. *(RNA splicing)*
The splicing reaction takes place in the nucleus of the cell prior to capping and polyadenylation as part of the post-transcriptional modification of eukaryotic RNA. U1 small nuclear ribonucleoprotein (snRNP) recognizes a 9 base-pair region of the introns involved and is thought to precipitate the organized formation of the large particle termed the spliceosome on the RNA. The splicing reaction then cuts the intron at the 5' end and forms a "lariat" structure by covalently binding the cut 5' end of the intron to a sequence on the 3' end. The intron is then cut again at the 3' end and thus is cut out of the RNA.

52. The answer is A. *(Carcinoid of the appendix)*
The most common tumor of the appendix is a carcinoid tumor. The neoplastic cells show neuroendocrine differentiation. The cells grow in nests and are associated with a delicate, branching vascular network. The nuclei of the cells have a "salt and pepper" chromatin distribution. Typically, the cytoplasm of the cells contain granules, which are visible by special stains. Silver salts turn the granules black, thus they are argyrophilic. The behavior of these tumors is related to their depth of invasion into the muscular wall and serosal adipose tissue.

53. The answer is D. *(Antioxidants)*
Transketolase is a part of the nonoxidative phase of the hexose monophosphate shunt and has no known role in protecting red blood cells from oxygen insult. A number of enzymes are involved in the protection of red blood cells from oxygen insult by hydrogen peroxide. Glutathione peroxidase catalyzes the reduction of hydrogen peroxide to water. The reduced nicotinamide-adenine dinucleotide phosphate (NADPH) utilized by glutathione reductase to regenerate reduced glutathione is produced in the 6-phosphogluconate dehydrogenase reaction. Catalase results in the decomposition of hydrogen peroxide to water and molecular oxygen.

54. The answer is D. *(Immunology; Arthus reaction)*
The Arthus reaction requires relatively large amounts of antibody and antigen, which then form insoluble complexes and begin to accumulate endogenously. When the aggregates are large enough, the complement cascade is activated. The formation of complement fragments C3a and C5a causes an increase in vascular permeability with resulting edema. Neutrophils and platelets accumulate at the site of the reaction. The activated neutrophils release a host of proteases and collagenases, resulting in rupture of the vessel wall, hemorrhage, and local necrosis. Serum sickness is the most common type III reaction, and the Arthus reaction is the least common.

55. The answer is D. *(Mechanism of action of zidovudine and treatment of AIDS)*
Zidovudine (ZDV) is currently the most important agent available for the palliation of AIDS. ZDV is phosphorylated to a deoxynucleoside derivative, which inhibits viral RNA-dependent DNA polymerase. Its selectivity is a function of its specificity for reverse transcriptase compared to human DNA polymerase. Granulocytopenia and anemia occur in up to 45% of treated patients, and resistance does occur to the drug after prolonged therapy. ZDV delays the development of signs and symptoms of AIDS in patients who are asymptomatic and improves the clinical symptoms of patients with AIDS at most stages in their disease. Thus, the incidence of opportunistic infections decreases, and there are some improvements in neurologic deficits, AIDS-associated thrombocytopenia, psoriasis, and lymphocytic interstitial pneumonia.

56. The answer is B. *(Vascular permeability; inflammation)*
Eosinophil chemotactic factor (ECF) is a set of tetrapeptides that produces a chemotactic gradient to attract eosinophils but has no effect on vascular permeability. Histamine and serotonin increase vascular permeability by causing post-capillary venular contraction. Slow-reacting substance of anaphylaxis (leukotrienes C_4 and D_4) are the only eicosanoids that directly increase vascular permeability. Both serotonin and slow-reacting substance of anaphylaxis increase vascular permeability.

57. The answer is E. *(Chronic obstructive pulmonary disease)*
Risk for chronic obstructive pulmonary disease (COPD) with various degrees of emphysema or chronic bronchitis is strongly associated with cigarette smoking and exposure to irritating substances in the environment (e.g., sulfur dioxide) or workplace (e.g., silica, cotton or grain dust, toluene diisocyanate). Usually, it is associated with older age-groups, especially individuals with preexisting lung disease. A genetically linked deficiency in α_1-antitrypsin is strongly linked to premature obstructive pulmonary disease. Although intravenous drug abuse is associated with pulmonary complications, including acute respiratory failure and opportunistic infections accompanying immunodeficiency-like syndromes in certain individuals, it is not usually considered a risk factor for COPD.

58. The answer is B. *(Nitrogen metabolism)*
Negative nitrogen balance would result from defective cholecystokinin-pancreozymin (CCK-PZ) production when the consumption of dietary protein is normal. Negative nitrogen balance occurs when the excretion of nitrogen exceeds the intake of nitrogen. A number of conditions can cause a negative nitrogen balance, including a deficiency in any one of the essential amino acids or a defect in the intestinal phase of protein digestion and absorption. CCK-PZ is essential for stimulating the secretion of inactive pancreatic zymogens, which become active proteases in the small intestine. The intestinal phase of digestion is essential to maintaining nitrogen balance; the gastric phase appears to have little, if any, impact. For example, gastric resection can be performed without affecting nitrogen balance. In phenylketonuria (PKU), tyrosine becomes an essential amino acid and must be supplied in the diet.

59. The answer is C. *(Human genetics and Duchenne muscular dystrophy)*
In Duchenne muscular dystrophy (DMD) the amount of dystrophin (a 400-kilodalton protein of unknown function but thought to be involved in Ca^{2+} regulation) is reduced from its normal 0.002% of total protein. Derangement of Ca^{2+} homeostasis is thought to be the cause of the excessive shortening of the sarcomeres. The affected muscle groups hypertrophy due to replacement of muscle mass by fibrofatty tissue. DMD is most often transmitted from a female carrier to the affected male (about 1 per 3500 liveborn males) by X-linked recessive inheritance (myotonic dystrophy is associated with mutations on chromosome 19), although approximately one-third of the cases appear to be due to spontaneously arising mutations.

60. The answer is D. *(Virulence factors; group A streptococci)*
The symptoms and clinical microbiology results indicate that the child has scarlet fever caused by a group A streptococcus *(Streptococcus pyogenes)* infection. This organism causes hemolysis by producing

extracellular hemolysins such as streptolysin O. Other important virulence factors of this organism include membrane-bound protein (M protein) [which is antiphagocytic and also helps mediate adhesion], lipoteichoic acid (which also mediates adhesion), and a hyaluronic acid capsule. The erythrogenic toxins responsible for scarlet fever rash are not hemolytic.

61. The answer is E. *(Protein synthesis)*
The synthetic polynucleotide sequence of CAACAACAACAA... could be read by the in vitro protein synthesizing system starting at the first C, the first A, or the second A. In the first case, the first triplet codon would be CAA, which codes for glutamine. In the second case, the first triplet codon would be AAC, which codes for asparagine; and in the last case, the first triplet codon would be ACA, which codes for threonine.

62–63. The answers are: 62-A, 63-C. *(Biostatistics)*
The variables described in the question are continuous in that their values are along a continuum as are age and IQ, as opposed to being categorical. Categorical variables, such as sex, race, and marital status, require the use of nonparametric statistical tests, such as the chi-squared test.

A null hypothesis is the hypothesis that an observed difference is due to chance alone and not to a systematic cause. In the study question, the null hypothesis is that there is no relationship between temperature and body weight. The study is designed to disprove the null hypothesis. The null hypothesis does not involve a *P* value, although a cutoff is generally chosen to show the likelihood that an association between variables is not due to chance alone (i.e., $P = 0.05$ means that there is a 5% probability that the two events or measurements are similar due to chance alone).

64. The answer is E. *(Bacterial pigment production)*
Pseudomonas aeruginosa, Staphylococcus aureus, and *Serratia marcescens* are all pigment producers. Pigment production by bacteria is associated with both gram-positive and gram-negative organisms. *P. aeruginosa* and *S. marcescens* produce endotoxins, and only *S. aureus* produces enterotoxin and lipoteichoic acids. None of the organisms listed produce mycolic acids.

65. The answer is B. *(Mycobacteria)*
Mycobacterium tuberculosis produces factors such as sulfatides, which inhibit the fusion of phagosomes with lysosomes. In addition to inhibiting phagosome–lysosome fusion, *M. tuberculosis* escapes engulfment by lysosomes. The organisms are also resistant to phagocytic killing because of their tough cell surface.

66. The answer is B. *(Autonomic pharmacology and effects of antimuscarinic agents)*
Atropine may abolish the parasympathetic input that normally maintains a relatively slow heart rate. Indeed, atropine is often used intraoperatively (and in emergencies) to increase heart rate. Atropine inhibits secretions from salivary, lacrimal, bronchial, and sweat glands. It causes mydriasis and cycloplegia. It has no effect on skeletal muscle, in which neuromuscular transmission involves acetylcholine (ACh) and nicotinic, not muscarinic, receptors.

67. The answer is B. *(G proteins and signal transduction)*
Guanosine triphosphate (GTP)–binding proteins (G proteins) are involved with the process of signal transduction and are the target of toxins, such as pertussis and cholera toxins. G proteins are activated when bound to GTP and deactivate via the hydrolysis of GTP to form guanosine diphosphate (GDP).

68. The answer is D. *(Bronchioloalveolar carcinoma)*
Bronchioloalveolar carcinomas are well differentiated adenocarcinomas, which grow in a nondestructive fashion over the matrix of the alveolar septa, replacing normal pneumocytes. This pattern has been called lepidic growth. Bronchioloalveolar carcinomas also have a propensity for aerogenous and lymphatic spread, and widespread intrapulmonary metastases may occur.

69. The answer is E. *(Cushing's syndrome)*
Cushing's syndrome may be caused by hypothalamic or pituitary pathology or both, adrenal adenoma (or carcinoma), and exogenous glucocorticoid administration. In pediatric cases, severe growth retardation may occur before closure of the epiphysis during puberty. Hypersecretion of adrenocorticotropic hormone (ACTH) from the pituitary gland, due to either an underlying tumor or overstimulation from corticotropin releasing factor (CRF) of hypothalamic origin, stimulates the adrenal cortex to release excessive amounts of glucocorticoids (and mineralocorticoids). Other sites of excessive ACTH secretion, including tumors of nonendocrine origin, may be important. A useful initial screen to detect the presence

of the syndrome is to inject dexamethasone and then to monitor the expected suppression of cortisol (due to pituitary inhibition) in plasma the following day. Patients with various forms of Cushing's syndrome and a responsive adrenal cortex will not undergo the predicted suppression until considerably higher amounts of dexamethasone are administered. Subsequent tests [including urinary secretion and administration of metyrapone (cortisol synthesis inhibitor)] and diagnostic procedures will help to identify the source of the excessive cortisol production.

70. The answer is D. *(Therapeutic effects in neoplasia)*
Paradoxically, patients with histologically "unfavorable" high-grade lymphomas show long-term survival if a complete clinical remission can be attained. However, it is rare to attain cure in histologically low-grade "favorable" non-Hodgkin's lymphomas: Patients die gradually from bone marrow compromise or lymphoma over many years. Long-term survival after 5 years for diffuse large cell lymphomas is roughly 50%. Those who do not attain complete remission usually die within several years. Spontaneous remissions are rarely seen in aggressive lymphomas.

71–75. The answers are: 71-D, 72-A, 73-C, 74-E, 75-C. *(Diabetes mellitus)*
The beta cells of the islets of Langerhans are the major site of insulin production in the pancreas. In insulin-dependent diabetes mellitus (IDDM), these cells are affected by genetic, autoimmune, viral, or other environmental factors so that they produce inadequate or no insulin.

Patients with type I IDDM are often started on daily injections of an intermediate-acting insulin preparation. Oral hypoglycemic agents such as glipizide are contraindicated in this group. Although abstinence from carbohydrates was initially thought appropriate, dietary manipulations now generally involve maintaining a complex carbohydrate diet with an emphasis on minimizing the intake of fats, especially saturated fats. Exercise is useful in an attempt to normalize peripheral tissue sensitivity to exogenous insulin.

Alpha cells of the endocrine pancreas secrete glucagon that increases blood glucose by increasing glycogenolysis and gluconeogenesis in the liver. Growth hormone (GH) opposes the action of insulin by interfering with the body's ability to use glucose. Somatostatin suppresses glucagon secretion and, therefore, tends to decrease blood glucose.

In spite of control of blood glucose levels with exogenous insulin, diet, and exercise in patients with IDDM, chronic changes in the microcirculation (especially in the kidney and eye) and macrocirculation (e.g., atherosclerosis) frequently occur. In addition, peripheral polyneuropathy is the most common diabetic neuropathy noted and appears to be associated with accumulation of sorbitol within Schwann cells. Currently, there is no association of IDDM and pulmonary hypertension.

Diabetic ketoacidosis is a common problem, and coma may ensue in 10% of the individuals. Rapid deep breathing (Kussmaul's respiration) is an important sign of such ketoacidosis and is the result of compensatory mechanisms in response to metabolic acidosis. In patients with hypoglycemic coma (from exuberant effects of insulin), a history of a skipped meal or vigorous exercise is helpful. In addition, their coma is often accompanied by profuse sweating rather than dehydration (which may be the case in ketoacidosis). Obviously, discerning between the two causes is critical to establish appropriate emergency therapy, and blood glucose levels will confirm clinical impressions.

76. The answer is E. *(Characteristics of volatile anesthetics)*
Halothane and methoxyflurane are typical inhalational drugs, which tend to depress both the cardiovascular and respiratory systems. Methoxyflurane is more potent (i.e., it has a lower minimal alveolar concentration) than halothane, as predicted from its higher oil:gas partition coefficient. Both result in considerably slower induction than nitrous oxide since their respective blood:gas partition coefficients are greater than that of nitrous oxide. Similarly, recovery from methoxyflurane is slower than that from halothane since its oil:gas partition coefficient is greater than that of halothane. An increase in ventilatory rate will make the onset of anesthesia more rapid for all inhalational anesthetics.

77. The answer is E. *(Protein synthesis)*
Protein synthesis occurs in both the cytoplasm and the mitochondria of cells and requires large amounts of energy. In addition to requiring adenosine triphosphate (ATP) for the formation of aminoacyl transfer RNA (tRNA), guanosine triphosphate (GTP) is required for initiation, formation, translocation, and termination of the peptide bond. Protein synthesis requires messenger RNA (mRNA), tRNA, and ribosomal RNA (rRNA). Peptide-bond formation involves the transfer of the nascent polypeptide chain from one tRNA to the amino group of another aminoacyl tRNA. This reaction is accomplished by the enzyme complex known as peptidyltransferase, which is an integral part of the 50S ribosomal subunits.

78. The answer is B. *(DNA and restriction enzymes)*
Restriction enzymes recognize specific base sequences in double-helical DNA and cleave both strands of the duplex at specific sites. Most of the cleavage sites contain a twofold rotational symmetry (the recognized sequence is palindromic). The cuts resulting from these enzymes may be either staggered or blunt. Restriction enzymes can cleave DNA molecules into a number of specific fragments. These enzymes are specific for DNA; they do not cleave RNA.

79. The answer is C. *(Physician–patient interactions)*
Regular, structured visits by the nurses can help to reassure a dependent and frightened patient and keep the nurses from feeling resentful. The patient's disease and disability have made him feel angry and out of control, and he is acting out his feelings by bothering the nurses. Punitive actions and indirect warfare with the patient will not remedy the situation.

80. The answer is C. *(Osteoclasts; bone metabolism)*
Osteoclasts are stimulated by parathyroid hormone and inhibited by calcitonin. Osteoclasts are multinucleated cells found on the surface of bone, often in Howship's lacuna. They are bone-resorbing cells involved in remodeling bone and in calcium homeostasis, and probably are derived from the macrophage–monocyte system.

81. The answer is C. *(Suicide risk)*
Elderly males have the highest suicide rate of any age-group, especially with the additional risk factors of widowerhood, alcohol abuse, chronic medical problems, and living alone. While renal insufficiency, silent myocardial infarction, peripheral neuropathy, and pneumonia are valid concerns, suicide has the highest lethal potential and need for active monitoring.

82. The answer is C. *(Antibacterial drug use during pregnancy)*
High levels of amoxicillin in the urine can be achieved because penicillins are eliminated mainly unmetabolized via the kidney. There is minimal risk for the fetus using this or other penicillins, although these agents do cross the placental barrier. Sulfonamides should be avoided due to displacement of bilirubin from serum albumin and resultant deposition of bilirubin in the central nervous system (CNS) [kernicterus] of the fetus and newborn, who do not yet have an intact blood–brain barrier. Minocycline should be avoided since tetracyclines are possibly teratogenic and can cause altered bone growth due to high calcium binding. Gentamicin can damage the eighth nerve in the fetus, leading to hearing impairment.

83. The answer is C. *(Antibiotic action)*
Chloramphenicol is bacteriostatic and, therefore, was responsible for the leveling off of *curve A.* All of the agents listed, except chloramphenicol, are bactericidal. Cephalothin, methicillin, and vancomycin all interfere with cell wall synthesis, leading to bursting and to cell death. Polymyxin affects cell membrane function, causing irreversible loss of small molecules from the cell. Chloramphenicol inhibits protein synthesis and is bacteriostatic. Hence, the cell number in the culture with chloramphenicol does not decrease, and the organisms are viable. Removal of chloramphenicol will result in growth.

84. The answer is C. *(Acid–base balance)*
According to the Henderson-Hasselbalch equation, the patient's pH is approximately 7.4 (normal), and his Pco_2 and $[HCO_3^-]$ are elevated. The elevation in Pco_2 (respiratory acidosis) has been compensated (i.e., normal pH) by a rise in $[HCO_3^-]$. This latter phenomenon is brought about by the kidneys excreting more acid and reabsorbing more HCO_3^-. Full compensation as in this example is most likely to be associated with chronic perturbations in acid–base balance. Such changes may be common in chronic obstructive pulmonary disease (COPD).

85. The answer is D. *(Immunologic disorders)*
Graves' disease is a thyroid disorder, but it is not known to be associated with thymomas. Thymomas, 90% of which are benign, are associated with myasthenia gravis, systemic lupus erythematosus, hypogammaglobulinemia, neutrophil agranulocytosis, and polymyositis. The significance of the association with these diseases, in particular myasthenia gravis, remains obscure, although removal of the thymus sometimes leads to regression of this disease.

86. The answer is B. *(Na^+ transport; adenosine triphosphate production)*
The ability of erythrocytes to pump Na^+ from the cytoplasm depends on a source of adenosine triphosphate (ATP). All of the erythrocyte's ATP is generated by glycolysis. The compound 1,3-diphosphoglycerate is a high-energy glycolytic intermediate that is converted to 3-phosphoglycerate with

the concomitant phosphorylation of adenosine diphosphate (ADP) to ATP. This reaction is catalyzed by phosphoglycerate kinase. Pyruvate carboxylase and glucose 6-phosphatase are gluconeogenic enzymes and are not present in the erythrocyte. Malate dehydrogenase is a mitochondrial enzyme and is not present in the erythrocyte. Stearoyl coenzyme A (CoA) desaturase is an enzyme in β-oxidation and is not present in the erythrocyte.

87. The answer is C. *(Human immunodeficiency virus)*
The human immunodeficiency virus (HIV) has a demonstrated ability to infect any cell with a CD4 receptor, which includes T-helper cells, macrophages, and a subset of brain cells. The virus particle attaches to the cell via the CD4 receptor and gains entry through membrane fusion; it does not require endocytosis. During the replication process, a large amount of viral glycoprotein is produced, which becomes integrated into the host cell membrane. This can either lead to a budding of new virus or fusion with another uninfected CD4$^+$ cell. One infected cell can fuse in this fashion with a large number of uninfected cells, rendering them immunologically inactive.

88. The answer is B. *(Biostatistics)*
A paired t-test allows a comparison of mean K$^+$ values before and after treatment by comparing each patient's initial serum level to his or her repeat value.

89. The answer is E. *(Chlamydia trachomatis)*
Chlamydia trachomatis cannot synthesize adenosine triphosphate (ATP) or oxidize the reduced form of nicotinamide-adenine dinucleotide (NADH) and is an obligate intracellular parasite. *C. trachomatis* organisms are internalized by host cells but evade destruction by preventing lysosomal fusion with the phagosome. *C. trachomatis* infections can be treated with tetracyclines, erythromycin, sulfonamides, sulfamethoxazole-trimethoprim, or rifampin.

90–91. The answers are: 90-D, 91-A. *(Differential diagnosis of infectious mononucleosis)*
This patient presents with the classic picture of infectious mononucleosis due to Epstein-Barr virus (EBV) infection. Extreme fatigue, difficulty concentrating, and fever are generalized systemic symptoms. Pharyngitis reflects the local immunologic response by T cells reactive against viral antigens on infected tonsillar B cells. Splenomegaly is also a consequence of immunologic response to EBV. Morphologic examination of lymphocytosis in the peripheral blood should reveal atypical lymphocytes, which are activated T cells with increased cytoplasm and less mature nuclear chromatin. Lymphocytes of infectious lymphocytosis and pertussis are morphologically normal, albeit increased in number; also pertussis is a disease of young children. Serum from this patient should yield a positive test for heterophile antibodies. The combination of pharyngitis and lymphadenopathy are characteristic of EBV-associated mononucleosis. Cytomegalovirus (CMV) mononucleosis lacks both of these features. Toxoplasmosis, a rare cause of mononucleosis, may have lymphadenopathy but not pharyngitis.

A not uncommon feature of infectious mononucleosis with EBV-mediated expansion of B cells is the development of antibodies to red cells, usually directed against the Ii antigen system. Most such antibodies are cold agglutinins; that is, they react with erythrocytes at temperatures less than 37° C. Cold agglutinins are usually of the immunoglobulin M (IgM) class, and a Coombs' test may or may not be positive. The virus-associated hemophagocytic syndrome has been seen in patients with EBV infections, although usually in immunocompromised patients. Direct infection of erythroid precursors is not a feature of EBV infection. Disseminated intravascular coagulation is a rare occurrence in infectious mononucleosis, and thrombocytopenia may cause petechiae but not hemorrhagic blood loss.

92. The answer is C. *(Replication cycle of viruses)*
During the eclipse phase, it is impossible to recover the virus particles from infected cells. The eclipse phase of the virus replication cycle is the final stage of adsorption (during which the virus invades the cell, multiplies, kills, and lyses the cell) and the process of penetration and uncoating (during which the virus particles become engulfed by the cytoplasm of the host cell where virus particles are broken down and released).

93. The answer is E. *(Cell function; organelles)*
Catalase is an enzyme that catalyzes the synthesis and degradation of hydrogen peroxide. Peroxisomes, also called microsomes, contain large amounts of catalase and, therefore, can be visualized after staining for catalase. Peroxisomes function in the metabolism of hydrogen peroxide, cholesterol, and lipids.

94. The answer is D. *(Delayed-type hypersensitivity reactions)*
The reaction observed was most likely caused by CD4$^+$ T cells. It is a delayed reaction, demonstrating that the T cells are working fine; therefore, the patient could neither lack all T-cell–mediated immune function nor suffer from DiGeorge syndrome. Sensitization has already occurred, so the secondary exposure would show symptoms faster than the primary reaction.

95–97. The answers are: 95-C, 96-C, 97-D. *(Open-angle glaucoma)*
Primary open-angle glaucoma is a genetically determined disorder that is the most common form of glaucoma in the general population. In the patient described in the question, a decreased outflow facility resulted in an imbalance between aqueous humor inflow and outflow. Outflow of aqueous humor is accomplished primarily by filtration through the trabecular network to the canal of Schlemm and, to a lesser extent, via absorption into iris blood vessels (uveoscleral outflow).

Cholinomimetics contract the ciliary muscle, thereby reducing resistance of aqueous humor outflow through the trabecular mesh and canal of Schlemm. Accordingly, topical administration of pilocarpine is the agent of choice for this problem. Atropine is a muscarinic antagonist and may exacerbate this problem. Succinylcholine is a depolarizing muscle relaxant and may exacerbate this condition by acutely contracting the accessory striated muscles of the eye prior to its paralyzing effects. Dexamethasone is a glucocorticoid that may exacerbate primary open-angle glaucoma by further reducing aqueous outflow via the trabecular meshwork. Tubocurarine is a nondepolarizing muscle relaxant that has relatively little effect on muscarinic receptors of the ciliary muscle.

Cholinesterase inhibitors, such as echothiophate are useful for glaucoma therapy but are well absorbed from the eye, and adverse systemic effects secondary to an increase in cholinergic activity are possible. Bronchoconstriction, especially in patients with hyperreactive airways, is a serious concern. In addition, these agents may promote micturition, increased gastrointestinal motility, decreased heart rate, and increased sweating — all physiologic responses typical of cholinomimetic effects secondary to inhibition of acetylcholinesterase.

98. The answer is C. *(Histopathology of peripheral nerve tumors)*
Schwannomas, such as neurilemomas, are solitary encapsulated tumors that form eccentric masses derived from peripheral nerves. The histologic appearance in the photomicrograph reveals Antoni A areas *(at right)*, which are cellular regions with spindle cells that have elongated tapered nuclei. These nuclei may palisade to form a picket fence–like array called a Verocay body. The looser, edematous zones with hyalinized blood vessels are called Antoni B areas. In contrast, neurofibromas form unencapsulated, onion-like, bulbous expansions of the nerve and are composed of loose interlacing bands of spindle cells with wavy nuclei.

99. The answer is A. *(Viral immunity)*
Antibodies cannot displace attached viruses from the host cell. The role of antibodies in preventing diseases caused by viruses is demonstrated by the effectiveness of the polio vaccine. For the poliovirus, and other viruses as well, antibodies bind to proteins on the surface of the viruses, which inhibits the virus from entering host cells. This attachment of immunoglobulins [most notably immunoglobulin G (IgG)] to the virus particle also leads to phagocytosis by attachment of the Fc portion of the antibody to macrophages. Attachment of the antibody to an infected host cell presenting viral antigens leads to complement-mediated lysis. Antibodies have been found that inhibit critical viral enzyme functions, such as neuraminidase of the influenza virus.

100. The answer is C. *(Gastrointestinal transport of fats)*
The formation of fatty acids and monoglyceride by pancreatic lipase is an important step in the digestive fate of triglycerides. Although there are gastric lipases, they have a relatively insignificant effect on ingested neutral fats. This is in contrast to a critical role for pancreatic lipase in the pancreatic juice. Neutral fats are emulsified by bile salts, and further agitation within the intestine makes their surface available for significant hydrolysis by the water-soluble pancreatic lipase. The products, fatty acids and 2-monoglyceride, would quickly convert back to fat if they were not made into micelles by bile salts. These bile salts ferry the micelles to the intestinal brush border where the hydrophobic fatty acid (and monoglyceride) rapidly diffuse passively through the lipid membrane.

101. The answer is E. *(Cholesterol biosynthesis)*
The synthesis of cholesterol utilizes acetyl coenzyme A (CoA) as the sole source of carbon atoms and reduced nicotinamide-adenine dinucleotide phosphate (NADPH) as a source of reducing equivalents. The NADPH is supplied primarily through two reactions, which are catalyzed by a glucose 6-phosphate dehydrogenase and 6-phosphogluconate dehydrogenase. The formation of 3-hydroxy-3-methylglutaryl

CoA (HMG CoA) results from the condensation of acetoacetyl CoA and acetyl CoA. The step that is committed to cholesterol synthesis is the conversion of HMG CoA to mevalonic acid. This step is catalyzed by HMG CoA reductase. HMG CoA is used to synthesize activated isoprenoid units, which are subsequently condensed to form squalene. Squalene is converted to lanosterol and then to cholesterol by a series of reactions that involve the addition of oxygen, cyclization to give the sterol ring structure, and elimination of three carbon atoms as carbon dioxide. Mevinolin is an inhibitor of HMG CoA reductase.

102. The answer is A. *(Neurophysiology)*
The anterior spinocerebellar tract is thought to cross the spinal cord and ascend to the cerebellum where it crosses the spinal cord again. The spinal thalamic tract crosses the cord only once. The cuneocerebellar tract contains fibers that run from the nucleus gracillus and cuneatus to the ipsilateral cerebellar hemisphere. The vestibulospinal tract also remains ipsilateral.

103. The answer is B. *(Epilepsy)*
The patient most likely has temporal lobe epilepsy, in which seizures are sometimes preceded by acoustic or olfactory hallucinations. Patients are also confused or anxious and sometimes perform complex and bizarre behaviors with no recall of events after the attack. Klüver-Bucy syndrome results from bilateral destruction of the temporal lobes and manifests as loss of fear and anger as well as docility, increased appetite, and hypersexuality. Jacksonian seizures are the classic tonic–clonic convulsions due to focal activity in the primary motor cortex. Petit mal (or absence) seizures usually occur in children and involve either brief myoclonic jerks, sudden loss in body tone with rapid recovery, or brief losses of consciousness during which the patient stares into space.

104. The answer is C. *(Enteric infection by enterotoxigenic bacteria)*
The symptoms of cholera result from the attachment of *Vibrio cholerae* to the intestinal mucosa and production of cholera toxin. The infection is acute, and the bacteria remain extracellular. The action of cholera toxin involves elevation of intestinal cyclic adenosine monophosphate (cAMP) levels, which results in massive fluid loss (seen as diarrhea).

105. The answer is B. *(Blood pressure regulation)*
Angiotensin-converting enzyme (ACE) hydrolyzes the decapeptide angiotensin I to the vasoconstrictor octapeptide, angiotensin II. Inhibition of this enzyme by a number of competitive antagonists is a new and useful way to lower blood pressure in some individuals. In addition to reducing circulating levels of the endogenous angiotensin II peptide, inhibition of ACE may have central effects, including a decrease in the dipsogenic effect of angiotensin II. Furthermore, angiotensin II appears to facilitate neurotransmission in the central and peripheral sympathetic nervous systems. Although angiotensin II is a potent stimulator of aldosterone secretion in the zona glomerulosa of the adrenal cortex, and inhibition of this effect might be expected to reduce blood pressure (by enhancing Na^+ excretion by the kidneys), there usually is little change in aldosterone levels because other endogenous secretagogues, including steroids, K^+, and minimal levels of angiotensin II, can maintain aldosterone secretion. Nonetheless, there is little indication to believe that the aldosterone level would actually increase, and if it did, this would result in Na^+ reabsorption, water retention, and an increase in arterial blood pressure.

106. The answer is C. *(Cell cycle; organelles)*
Centrioles are made of nine tubular triplets, and they function in mitotic spindle formation and in the production of cilia and flagella. Centrioles are self-duplicated in the S (synthesis) phase of the cell cycle.

107. The answer is B. *(Energy storage and transfer)*
A high-energy bond is defined as a bond that, when hydrolyzed, will release a sufficient amount of energy to drive the synthesis of adenosine triphosphate (ATP) from adenosine diphosphate (ADP) and inorganic phosphate (P_i). This requires approximately 7.3 kcal/mol. There are two intermediates in glycolysis that are high-energy compounds: phosphoenolpyruvate and 1,3-bisphosphoglycerate. In the tricarboxylic acid (TCA) cycle, the conversion of succinyl coenzyme A (CoA) to succinate releases enough energy to synthesize guanosine triphosphate (GTP) from guanosine diphosphate (GDP) and P_i. In muscle tissue, phosphocreatine is a storage form of high energy. The hydrolysis of phosphate from phosphocreatine is coupled with the synthesis of ATP. A reaction that is exergonic is accompanied by a $\Delta G°$ that is < 0. The relationship between $\Delta G°$ and K_{eq} is $\Delta G° = -RT \ln K_{eq}$. For a reaction to proceed spontaneously, the K_{eq} must be > 1 and the $\Delta G°$ must be < 0.

108. The answer is B. *(Oxidative enzymes)*
The extraction of β-hydroxybutyrate from blood, and its oxidation to carbon dioxide and water, requires the participation of acetoacetate thiokinase and β-hydroxybutyrate dehydrogenase. All tissues except the liver use β-hydroxybutyrate as a metabolic fuel. The enzymes required for catabolism of the ketone bodies are localized in the mitochondria. These enzymes are: β-hydroxybutyrate dehydrogenase; succinyl coenzyme A (CoA); acetoacetate acyltransferase; and acetoacetate thiokinase. 3-Hydroxy-3-methylglutaryl CoA (HMG CoA) lyase catalyzes a step in fatty acid oxidation that takes place in the kidneys or liver. HMG CoA lyase breaks down *(S)*-3-hydroxy-3-methylglutaryl CoA into acetyl CoA and acetoacetate.

109–111. The answers are: 109-B, 110-E, 111-B. *(Thiazide diuretic therapy)*
The thiazide diuretics, such as hydrochlorothiazide, primarily act in the early distal tubules by binding to a membrane protein that is a Na^+ and Cl^- cotransporter. Thus, both Na^+ but more importantly Cl^- reabsorption in the early distal tubules is blocked. The thiazide diuretics also have a small effect in the late proximal tubules.

While most diuretics can cause all of the untoward effects listed in the question, the patient's neuromuscular dysfunction is most likely the result of hypokalemia, the most important and most serious side effect listed. Hypokalemia is produced because the diuretics cause a large amount of Na^+ to collect in the distal tubules, which leads to Na^+ reabsorption (sodium avidity) and a concomitant depletion of K^+. This Na^+–K^+ exchange site is a primary mechanism for renal control of K^+ homeostasis.

Because this patient is suffering from classic diuretic-induced K^+ loss, he should be supplemented with K^+. The physician may also prescribe a K^+-sparing diuretic, such as amiloride or spironolactone, to be used in combination with a reduced dosage of the thiazide diuretic to maintain K^+ balance. The altered blood K^+ would lead to an increased sensitivity to digitalis-related cardiovascular toxicity, so digitalis should not be used to treat this patient's edema.

112. The answer is D. *(Empiric antibacterial therapy in an immunocompromised host)*
The most likely diagnosis explaining the patient's condition is septic shock secondary to bacteremia. Chemotherapy for cancer is a common cause of neutropenia, with subsequent fever and infection. The risk is high when the white blood cell count is less than $500/\mu l$. In addition, cold, clammy skin is indicative of peripheral vascular shutdown. Lactic acid buildup will lead to metabolic acidosis and compensatory rapid breathing. Patients with neutropenic fever must be treated with double broad-spectrum antibacterial agents for gram-negative rods, including *Pseudomonas*. The combination of piperacillin, a broad-spectrum β-lactam, and gentamicin, an aminoglycoside, which has broad gram-negative activity, is a good choice. In addition, penicillin–aminoglycoside combinations may be synergistic because of the different mechanisms of action of these agents; penicillins are cell wall synthesis inhibitors, and aminoglycosides inhibit protein synthesis. Single aminoglycoside therapy with gentamicin or amikacin would not effectively prevent infection by resistant organisms. Both chloramphenicol and gentamicin are protein synthesis inhibitors and would not be expected to work synergistically.

113. The answer is A. *(Psychotherapy management)*
The patient motorically and nonverbally expresses (acts out) his conflictual feelings and anxiety about the closeness he feels towards his physician by avoiding a scheduled appointment. There is some degree of repression of these feelings, but the motor behavior indicates that the patient is acting out. Suppression is a *conscious* decision to postpone something, but missing these appointments was not done consciously.

114. The answer is C. *(Disaccharide structure and function)*
The structure shown is that of the milk disaccharide lactose. Lactose is composed of 1 mol of galactose and 1 mol of glucose, which are joined by a β-galactosidic linkage. Lactose is the substrate for the intestinal enzyme lactase, which hydrolyzes the disaccharide. Therefore, lactose would not be digested or absorbed by a lactase-deficient child. Since galactosemia arises from an impaired ability to metabolize galactose, lactose would not be a good source of calories for a child with galactosemia. Additional galactose would augment the problem. Since the only requirement for a reducing sugar is an unsubstituted carbonyl group, the disaccharide would give a positive result in the Fehling-Benedict reducing sugar test. The anomeric carbon of the glucose residue is in equilibrium with the open chain structure, thereby providing an unsubstituted carbonyl group.

115. The answer is C. *(Varicella-zoster virus)*
The lesions outside the dermatomal distribution are explained by depressed cell-mediated immunity. When varicella-zoster virus (VZV) goes outside a dermatomal distribution, it is because the affected person is immunosuppressed either from old age (> 65 years) or medication (in this case, chemotherapy).

Thymidine kinase-negative mutants rarely occur, except in human immunodeficiency virus (HIV) patients on prolonged prophylaxis with acyclovir. Initial exposure to the infection always leads to viral latency of the dorsal ganglia.

116. The answer is B. *(Histopathology of rheumatic fever)*
The photomicrograph of the heart shows an Aschoff body *(lower right)*, which is pathognomonic of a previous history of rheumatic fever, and the mitral stenosis is probably a consequence as well. Aschoff bodies constitute foci of fibrinoid necrosis surrounded by histiocytes, giant cells, and specialized histiocytes with linear chromatin called "caterpillar cells," which are seen with acute rheumatic fever and are eventually replaced by scar tissue. Tissue affected by rheumatic heart disease usually shows pericardial adhesions, valvular deformities, and fusion and shortening of the chordae tendineae.

117. The answer is A. *(Personality assessment)*
The major projective instrument of personality assessment is the Rorschach test. The thematic apperception test, sentence completion test, and projective drawings all are projective tests, but they are less well studied and yield more limited information. The Minnesota Multiphasic Personality Inventory, which is the most frequently used personality test, is an objective instrument, not a projective test.

118. The answer is C. *(Cell structure; membranes)*
The cell membrane is composed of a variety of proteins scattered within a phospholipid bilayer. The phospholipid molecules contain a hydrophilic head and a hydrophobic tail and, therefore, are amphipathic. The cell membrane readily allows the diffusion of molecules such as oxygen, carbon dioxide, nitrogen, and water; however, glucose does not diffuse through the cell readily, and entry into the cell is enhanced by carrier proteins (facilitated diffusion and active transport).

119. The answer is D. *(Cardiac mechanics and sounds)*
Pulmonary stenosis and pulmonary hypertension are associated with a prominent S_4 heart sound. Left-to-right shunts involving the left ventricle (e.g., ventricular septal defects and patent ductus arteriosus) are associated with a prominent S_3 heart sound, as are mitral regurgitation and left ventricular failure.

120. The answer is D. *(Tuberculosis culture; diagnostic tests)*
Isolation of *Mycobacterium tuberculosis* is diagnostic of active tuberculosis. The tuberculin test can be positive in the absence of active disease. The clinical findings are not specifically pathognomonic for tuberculosis, nor is demonstration of acid-fast organisms.

121. The answer is C. *(Prokaryotic and eukaryotic differences)*
Since shigellae are gram-negative prokaryotic bacteria, they have peptidoglycan-containing cell walls, lipopolysaccharide, 70S ribosomes, RNA, and DNA, but they do not have sterols in their plasma membranes. *Giardia* species are eukaryotic protozoa with 80S ribosomes, RNA, DNA, and sterol-containing plasma membranes.

122. The answer is D. *(Enzyme catalysis)*
The activation energy is the amount of energy required to pass into the transition state; the rate of the reaction depends on the number of molecules in the transition state. Increasing the activation energy lowers the reaction rate. Each enzyme has two kinetic parameters: V_{max} is an index of catalytic efficiency, and K_m is a measure of the affinity of the enzyme for the substrate. The binding of substrate to enzyme induces a conformational change in which the functional group that participates in catalysis is appropriately juxtaposed with the substrate bonds that are to be altered in the reaction. General acid–base catalysis is a catalytic mode frequently used by enzymes.

123. The answer is B. *(Tumor immunology)*
Antigens of physically induced tumors, such as those induced by chemical carcinogens, ultraviolet light, or x-rays, exhibit little or no antigenic cross-reactivity. Since random mutations are the most likely explanation for these types of tumors, each tumor displays distinct antigenic specificity. The cells of a given tumor arise from a single cell and are, therefore, antigenically similar.

124. The answer is E. *(Respiratory failure)*
Adult respiratory distress syndrome (ARDS) is a model of acute alveolar injury with pulmonary edema and respiratory failure. A number of conditions can lead to ARDS, particularly if high concentrations of oxygen are used as supportive respiratory therapy. Focal atelectasis and alveolar collapse occur with the development of pulmonary edema; hyaline membranes appear, type II pneumocytes proliferate, and

there is variable damage to the alveolar walls. The mechanisms of ARDS are not completely understood. The permeability of the endothelium of the pulmonary capillary and the epithelium of the alveolar wall is increased in ARDS, and it is responsible, in part, for the characteristics of the syndrome.

125. The answer is C. *(Anatomy of the respiratory system)*
Type II pneumocytes cover less than 5% of the alveolar surface, but they form a reserve for replacement of damaged type I pneumocytes. These multilamellar bodies are the source of the phospholipid-containing pulmonary surfactant. Defects in these cells contribute to infant and adult respiratory distress.

126. The answer is A. *(Hematopoietic–lymphoreticular system)*
Reed-Sternberg cells are diagnostic for Hodgkin's lymphoma. The Philadelphia chromosome and decreased quantities of leukocyte alkaline phosphatase are commonly observed in chronic myelogenous leukemia. Auer rods are most often seen in increased numbers in acute myelogenous or myelomonocytic leukemia.

127. The answer is E. *(Cellular signal transduction)*
The nuclear oncogene product c-*fos* assists in the regulation of gene expression. Although its expression is affected by second messengers, it is not thought of as a second messenger. Inositol 1,4,5-triphosphate (IP_3) and diacylglycerol (DAG) are important second messengers generated by phospholipase C from phosphatidylinositol biphosphate. IP_3 causes the release of intracellular stores of Ca^{2+}, which is also an important second messenger, and DAG activates a Ca^{2+}-dependent protein kinase, protein kinase C. Cyclic adenosine monophosphate (cAMP) is synthesized by adenylate cyclase from adenosine trophosphate (ATP) and can act as a second messenger to activate enzymes such as cAMP-dependent protein kinase.

128. The answer is B. *(Neurologic diagnosis)*
The selectivity of the deficit makes a supraforaminal lesion and a peripheral neuropathy impossible. We are not told if position sense is impaired: If it is, the posterior column of the spinal cord becomes a possibility, but an isolated vibratory deficit can occur as a normal aging change. The practical point is that when diminished vibratory sensation is encountered, position sense must be tested carefully to make the branch point.

129. The answer is D. *(Embolism)*
Thrombi from the left side of the heart to the parent vessels of the cerebral arteries all may embolize to occlude a cerebral artery; however, the abdominal aorta is beyond these vessels that lead to the brain and, thus, is unlikely to cause an embolism in the brain. Severe fracture of any long bone may result in a fat embolus to the cerebral arteries.

130. The answer is A. *(Autonomic pharmacology)*
Indirect-acting sympathomimetic agents, like amphetamine, are transported into nerve terminals by the uptake 1 mechanism where they displace norepinephrine to account for the pressor response. Because these agents lack hydroxyl groups on the catechol ring, they are without significant direct effects on synaptic receptors. Thus, their action is affected by the presence of other agents that modify adrenergic transmission. Reserpine depletes norepinephrine stores, and monoamine oxidase (MAO) inhibitors may potentiate norepinephrine levels. Thus, the pressor response to amphetamine would be potentiated by a MAO inhibitor and decreased by reserpine. Imipramine interferes with uptake of amphetamine and reduces its effect in this and other ways. A hallmark of indirect-acting sympathomimetics is tolerance or tachyphylaxis. This is presumably secondary to depletion of endogenous norepinephrine pools after repetitive application of amphetamine.

131. The answer is C. *(Nucleic acid transfer)*
Transduction is the technique whereby a virus, known as a bacteriophage, is used to introduce DNA into bacteria. Transformation uses high concentrations of calcium chloride to help DNA cross the bacterial plasma membrane. Conjugation refers to direct transfer of DNA between bacteria. Circular, or plasmid, DNA is the form of DNA most commonly used to transfer genes into bacteria via transformation.

132–138. The answers are: 132-D, 133-B, 134-E, 135-D, 136-C, 137-B, 138-C. *(Anatomy of skeletal muscles and properties of halothane)*
Unlike intravenous anesthetics (e.g., methohexital), inhalational anesthetics such as halothane do not possess notable excitatory effects on the central nervous system (CNS), and, thus, do not lower seizure

threshold. All anesthetics tend to depress cardiac function and respiratory drive. Halothane and other anesthetics may induce malignant hyperthermia in certain genetically susceptible individuals.

The anterior cruciate ligament (ACL) is important to the proper functioning of the knee joint. The ACL attaches the femur to the tibia. Damage to this ligament is usually sports-related and due to rapid deceleration or torque. The ligament is essential to the stability of the knee joint, and surgery is necessary to prevent further injury.

Latin for "little vinegar saucer," the acetabulum is the rounded cavity on the external surface of the innominate bone that receives the head of the femur.

The epiphyseal plate lies between the epiphysis and diaphysis of long bones and is the area of highest mitotic activity. During bone growth, the epiphyseal plates migrate distally, finally becoming epiphyseal lines when growth is completed.

The cuboid is a tarsal bone. The navicular is both a carpal and a tarsal bone. All of the other bones listed (i.e., capitate, trapezium, trapezoid) are carpal bones.

A haversian system, or osteon, is made up of osteocytes, lacunae, canaliculi, and concentric lamellae. It is the fundamental unit of compact bone. Compact bone is made up of lamellae, which are parallel bony columns that surround a central (haversian) canal; these canals are neurovascular channels and interconnect via Volkmann's canals. Osteocytes occupy lacunae and communicate with each other via gap junctions that are formed between tiny cytoplasmic projections found in canaliculi. Trabeculae are characteristic features of cancellous (spongy) bone.

139. The answer is C. *(Diagnostic tests)*
Lumbar puncture is absolutely contraindicated in patients with intracranial neoplasms because it may cause a rapid extrusion of brain tissue of the cerebral hemisphere through the tentorial notch or of the medulla and cerebellum through the foramen magnum. This is due to the fact that these tumors usually cause high cerebrospinal fluid (CSF) pressure buildup, and lumbar puncture allows rapid depressurization of the fluid. Computed tomography (CT) with contrast medium, nuclear magnetic resonance (NMR), and x-ray are all very useful tools in imaging brain tumors and do not cause the complications above.

140. The answer is A. *(Immunogobulin E–mediated hypersensitivity)*
The scientist has developed an allergy after repeated exposure to the rodent. The late symptom complex was induced by mast cells triggered by previous interaction of rodent antigen with immunoglobulin E (IgE). This is a typical late phase set of reactions, which are mast-cell mediated; no complement is involved. Corticosteroids will block the late reaction. The involvement of histamine is early, not late.

141. The answer is A. *(Renal physiology)*
If glomerular filtration decreases, excessive reabsorption of Na^+ (and Cl^-) will occur in the ascending limb of the loop of Henle. The decrease in ion concentration within the distal tubules causes the release of renin from the juxtaglomerular cells (*1*), with subsequent formation of angiotensin II and vasoconstriction of the efferent arteriole (*2*) to help return filtration to normal values. In addition, there will be afferent arteriolar vasodilation to support glomerular filtration.

142. The answer is D. *(Gram stain; bacterial growth)*
Bacterial spores probably caused the decrease in the number of cells expected from the turbidity of the culture. Spores contribute to turbidity, but they do not stain in Gram's procedure.

143. The answer is C. *(Hemodynamics)*
Under the circumstances described in the question, the stroke volume is 100 ml. Cardiac output is the ratio of oxygen consumption to the arteriovenous difference. In this case, it is:

$$\frac{300 \ ml/min}{20 \ ml/100 \ ml - 15 \ ml/100 \ ml} = 6000 \ ml/min$$

Stroke volume is the ratio of cardiac output to heart rate:

$$\frac{6000 \ ml/min}{60 \ min} = 100 \ ml$$

144. The answer is C. *(Antiphagocytic virulence factors)*
Opsonizing antibodies promote phagocytosis and are often directed against the capsules of pathogens, including *Streptococcus pneumoniae*. The most important function of the *S. pneumoniae* capsule is to inhibit phagocytosis (until opsonizing antibodies are produced). The capsules of both *Hemophilus influenzae* type B and *Neisseria meningitidis* are polysaccharides that elicit a poor T-cell–dependent immune

response. The existing DTP (diphtheria-tetanus-pertussis) vaccine contains killed whole *Bordetella pertussis* cells, not purified capsules.

145. The answer is D. *(Structure and function of proteins)*
The chemical properties of proteins are determined by the nature of the constituent amino acid side chains. There are no ionizing groups, physiologically speaking, on the side chain of serine to provide buffering capacity. Only those amino acids with aromatic side chains absorb significantly in the ultraviolet range. Both glutamic acid and aspartic acid have a pI of approximately 4.5, and only L-amino acids are incorporated into protein. The side chain of proline contains a cyclic ring that cannot bond hydrogen and, therefore, disrupts the α-helical structure.

146. The answer is D. *(Effects of exogenous testosterone)*
Although testosterone is required for normal spermatogenesis, it is involved in an important feedback inhibition pathway. Accordingly, introduction of high concentrations of testosterone can inhibit gonadatropin-releasing hormone production in the hypothalamus and interfere with important steps in spermatogenesis induced by leuteinizing hormone. In addition, testosterone can be metabolized to estrogens in men as well as women, and this estrogen formation can add to the inhibition of normal spermatogenesis. This effect is usually reversible in most mature men but can persist in a subset of anabolic steroid abusers. Testosterone is very likely to produce its well-known masculinization effects in mature women and can produce feminization in men. Although testosterone has a significant myotrophic effect on muscle mass in children, it is never used in this age-group because it causes closure of the epiphysis of long bones.

147. The answer is A. *(Diagnosis of myelodysplastic syndrome)*
Clinically persistent and unexplained cytopenias associated with morphologically abnormal differentiation in bone marrow precursors defines preleukemia, often referred to as the myelodysplastic syndrome. Many of these individuals will have bone marrow blast percentages of less than 5%, and patients suffer from complications of bone marrow failure such as bleeding, infection, and anemia. Others will show an increase in bone marrow blasts between 5% and 30% and have a higher propensity to develop frank acute myeloid leukemia, particularly at the higher levels. Bone marrow blasts greater than 30% define acute leukemia. Cytogenetic changes, if present in myelodysplastic syndrome, are similar to those observed with acute myeloid leukemia, such as an extra chromosome 8, loss of chromosomes 5 or 7, or loss of the long arm of chromosomes 5 or 7. Despite megaloblastoid morphologic changes, these patients do not resolve with treatment for megaloblastic anemia. It is rare for chronic myelogenous leukemia to present with a low white cell and platelet count and bone marrow dyspoiesis.

148. The answer is D. *(Collagen biosynthesis)*
The biosynthesis of collagen by fibroblasts involves hydroxylation of prolyl and lysyl residues. These reactions are catalyzed by distinct hydroxylases, which require molecular oxygen, α-ketoglutarate, Fe^{2+}, and ascorbate. Hydroxyproline confers stability on the triple helix. Glycosylation occurs by the addition of a disaccharide unit to specific hydroxylysyl residues. By the end of the hydroxylation and glycosylation reactions, the formation of the triple helix is completed and the procollagen molecule is secreted. Following secretion, the globular heads of procollagen are removed from the amino and carboxy terminal regions to produce tropocollagen, which then assembles into collagen fibers.

149. The answer is C. *(Receptors; histamine (H_2) receptor antagonists; toxicology therapy)*
Cimetidine, like most drugs, interacts with a specific receptor, the histamine (H_2) receptor. Mannitol is the osmotic diuretic used most frequently in the prevention and treatment of acute renal failure occurring in conditions such as cardiovascular surgery, trauma, and hemolytic transfusion reactions. Ethylenediaminetetraacetic acid (EDTA) and dimercaprol chelate heavy metals but do not need to interact directly with any receptor for their pharmacologic actions.

150. The answer is D. *(Hemoglobin–oxygen interaction)*
The affinity of hemoglobin A_1 ($\alpha_2\beta_2$) for oxygen is decreased by an increase in H^+ concentration (a decrease in pH), an increase in the P_{CO_2}, or by an increase in the concentration of 2,3-diphosphoglycerate (DPG). All of these conditions result in a shift of the oxygen saturation curve to the right. Fetal hemoglobin ($\alpha_2\gamma_2$) has a higher affinity for oxygen than adult hemoglobin ($\alpha_2\beta_2$) and consequently becomes saturated at a lower P_{O_2}.

151. The answer is A. *(RNA function)*
The synthesis of RNA in eukaryotes requires three different RNA polymerases; one each for the synthesis of messenger RNA (mRNA), ribosomal RNA (rRNA), and transfer RNA (tRNA). All of these RNAs are required for protein synthesis. The ribosome is a complex made up of approximately 75 proteins and several types of rRNA and is the site where mRNA and tRNAs come together to participate in protein synthesis. The triplet base codons for amino acids are contained in mRNA; tRNA contains a complementary anticodon, which promotes interaction between mRNA and tRNA during protein synthesis.

152. The answer is A. *(Musculature of the oral cavity)*
During deglutition, the levator veli palatini muscle raises the soft palate to seal the nasopharynx. Contraction of the palatoglossus elevates the base of the tongue and, with help from the palatopharyngeus muscle, closes the oropharyngeal isthmus behind the food bolus. The superior constrictor muscle helps raise the posterior portion of the pharynx over the bolus.

153. The answer is C. *(Side effects of neuroleptics)*
Akathisia, an extrapyramidal side effect of neuroleptics, causes restlessness and an urge to keep moving. The agitation in the man presented in the question seems more motoric than psychic, making worsening psychosis less likely. While hyperthyroidism causes hyperactivity, this patient has no other symptoms of thyroid disease. Restless legs syndrome is a sleep-related disorder, generally associated with nocturnal myoclonus. It is described as a creepy, crawly feeling in the legs at rest (especially when supine) that is relieved by walking.

154. The answer is B. *(Extracellular matrix production and chondroblasts)*
Chondroblasts are cartilage cells located deep in the perichondrium, the dense connective capsule that surrounds cartilage. As chondroblasts secrete an extracellular matrix rich in type II collagen and cartilage proteoglycan, they become surrounded by their own extracellular matrix and differentiate into chondrocytes. Both chondroblasts and chondrocytes are capable of cell division by mitosis. The endosteum is a layer of osteoblasts in bone. The periosteum is the outer connective tissue covering of bone.

155. The answer is B. *(Pathophysiology of idiopathic thrombocytopenic purpura)*
Idiopathic thrombocytopenic purpura (ITP) is most common in young women, and the usual presentation is of isolated thrombocytopenia without associated illness. Amegakaryocytic thrombocytopenia can occur, but it is much less common, especially in this age-group. Drug-induced thrombocytopenia is also possible but is unlikely in a healthy woman who has no reason to take medications. Patients with thrombasthenia are not thrombocytopenic, and aleukemic leukemia is unlikely to occur without other cytopenias.

156–161. The answers are: 156-C, 157-B, 158-A, 159-E, 160-D, 161-A. *(Exocrine pancreatic function)*
Elevated serum amylase is the single most important diagnostic finding for confirmation of acute pancreatitis. A serum amylase level threefold higher than normal virtually confirms the diagnosis.
Secretin is composed of 27 amino acids, is secreted by the mucosal cells of the duodenum, and promotes the secretion of pancreatic juice rich in electrolytes and water. Cholecystokinin is released by mucosal cells in the upper small intestine in response to peptones and fats. It is absorbed into the bloodstream and stimulates the pancreas to secrete large quantities of digestive enzymes.
Although neuronal control of pancreatic exocrine function is secondary to hormonal control, parasympathetic stimulation of pancreatic secretory activity occurs via vagal fibers, which release acetylcholine (ACh).
Secretin and cholecystokinin are secreted by the mucosa of the small intestine into the bloodstream. They exert their effects after entering the pancreatic circulation. Secretin is stored in an inactive form in the S cells of the duodenum and is released and activated in response to acid. It causes the pancreas to secrete copious amounts of bicarbonate ion (HCO_3^-), but unlike cholecystokinin, which is secreted in response to food, secretin does not significantly affect pancreatic enzyme secretion. The proteolytic enzymes are synthesized as proenzymes, inactive precursors that must be processed before they are active. Many proenzymes, including chymotrypsinogen, procarboxypeptidase, and prophospholipase, are activated by trypsin. Trypsinogen is activated by enterokinase.

162. The answer is C. *(Immunology; complement fixation)*
The complement fixation test is composed of sheep red blood cells (SRBC), antibodies to SRBC, and complement. The concentration of complement is limiting, and any loss of complement is preflected by

a decrease in the extent of SRBC lysis. This loss of complement could be caused during preincubation of the complement with an antigen–antibody complex not related to the SRBC, which would cause fixation and activation of the cascade. All or most of the complement would be consumed so that the introduction of SRBC does not result in lysis. In this case, since lysis did occur, the patient's serum possesses no complement-fixable [immunoglobulin G (IgG)] anti-influenza type A antibodies. A cross-reactive antibody has no bearing on the complement fixation test.

163. The answer is D. *(Pulmonary mechanics)*
Inspiration is an active process brought about by contraction of the diaphragm. This contraction results in increased chest volume, thereby lowering pleural and alveolar pressure and creating a gradient for the movement of air. At the end of inspiration, flow is zero and alveolar pressure equals atmospheric pressure. The difference between alveolar and pleural pressure is the recoil pressure of the lung, which is always greatest at higher lung volumes and, thus, is greater at the end of inspiration. During expiration, inspiratory muscles relax, and the elastic forces of the lungs compress alveolar gas, which raises alveolar pressure to values greater than atmospheric pressure and creates a pressure gradient to expel gas from the lung.

164. The answer is D. *(Hormone receptors; Addison's disease)*
Addison's disease is due to an overall atrophy of the adrenal cortex and is not related to an abnormality in hormone receptors. Many peptide hormone receptors are transmembrane proteins that may elicit their full biologic response when only a small fraction of the receptors are occupied by hormone. The specificity of the response of a particular cell or tissue is defined, at least in part, by the types of receptors localized on or in the cell. Some hormone receptors are desensitized by phosphorylation. Following phosphorylation, dissociation of the hormone from the receptor may occur without a corresponding decrease in the biologic response.

165. The answer is A. *(RNA processing)*
RNA processing occurs in two locations within cells. The most common site is the cell nucleoplasm, where the majority of RNA transcribed in the nucleus is spliced, capped, and polyadenylated. The other site is the mitochondria, each of which contains a ring of DNA that codes for two ribosomal RNA (rRNA) molecules, proteins, and all the transfer RNA (tRNA) required to synthesize the encoded proteins.

166. The answer is C. *(Urea metabolism; amino acid enzymes)*
The pathway by which the α-amino groups of the amino acids are incorporated into urea involves a number of transaminases that transfer the amino group from the amino acids to α-ketoglutarate, with the concomitant formation of glutamate. The glutamate is converted back to α-ketoglutarate and ammonium by the mitochondrial enzyme glutamate dehydrogenase. The ammonium produced in the reaction is the substrate for carbamoyl phosphate synthesis. This reaction constitutes the first step in urea biosynthesis.

167. The answer is C. *(Neurophysiology)*
Patients born without a corpus callosum show no neurologic defects. Only lesions introduced after the brain has developed would produce symptoms. The Romberg sign is indicative of cerebellar disease and has no bearing in this case.

168. The answer is D. *(Neuroanatomy)*
The subthalamus is located (not surprisingly) below the thalamus. It is an exceedingly complex area of the brain connected to many areas integrating motor control but is not connected with the cerebellum.

169. The answer is B. *(DNA replication)*
Topoisomerase enzymes are important for regulating the equilibrium between supercoiled and relaxed DNA. Okazaki fragments are annealed by the actions of a ligase, and the newly synthesized DNA is "proofread" by a subunit of DNA polymerase III. The RNA primer is required to initiate DNA synthesis and is thought to be synthesized by RNA polymerase.

170–172. The answers are: 170-A, 171-E, 172-A. *(Cystic fibrosis)*
Inheritance via autosomal recessive genetic transmission suggests that each parent must have been a carrier. Since the parents of the patient in question are disease-free, they are heterozygous; thus, their chances of having another child with cystic fibrosis is one in four, according to mendelian genetics.

A deficiency in pancreatic lipases reduces the absorption of fat-soluble vitamins (A, D, and K). Vitamin K is critically important in the synthesis of clotting factors II, VII, IX, and X, and a deficiency in vitamin

K leads to bleeding diatheses manifested by a prolonged prothrombin time. Vitamins B_6 and C are water soluble and are less likely to be affected by pancreatic lipase deficiency.

Although clinical improvement from respiratory infections in cystic fibrosis occurs without eradication of bacteria from sputum during antibiotic therapy, it is standard procedure to treat the readily identifiable microorganisms. The gram-positive and particularly difficult to eradicate gram-negative bacteria (e.g., *Pseudomonas aeruginosa*) are often cultured from sputum, and a common regimen includes a β-lactam antibiotic, such as gentamicin, with a gram-negative antibiotic, such as the third-generation cephalosporin, ceftazidime. *P. aeruginosa* is often resistant to nitrofurantoin or nalidixic acid. Pentamidine is used for the treatment of protozoal infections, such as *Pneumocystis carinii*. Rifampin and isoniazid are used in the therapy of tuberculosis.

173. The answer is C. *(Histopathology of alcohol-induced acute liver damage)*
The liver biopsy shows the typical features of alcohol-induced acute liver injury, which include steatorrhea, acute inflammation, and Mallory bodies. Mallory bodies are intracellular filamentous material believed to be related to prekeratin, which is normally produced by the liver. This injury to the liver is a direct effect of alcohol.

174. The answer is C. *(Neoplasia of the reproductive tract)*
Twenty-five percent of males in the United States have a tumor in the prostate gland. A prostatic tumor rarely occurs before age 40 years, but the incidence rises rapidly with advancing age. Seventy-five percent of prostatic tumors arise in the posterior lobe, are easily palpable, and, therefore, are detectable.

175–176. The answers are: 175-D, 176-D. *(Pheochromocytoma)*
The paroxysmal symptoms and detection of an abdominal mass within the adrenal gland are consistent with a diagnosis of pheochromocytoma, a relatively rare tumor of the chromaffin cells of the adrenal medulla. The cells of the adrenal cortex are generally not affected, although extra-adrenal chromaffin cells are often involved.

Pharmacotherapy to manage the clinical symptoms includes the use of an α-adrenergic receptor blocker (phenoxybenzamine) either alone or in combination with a β-blocker. β-blockers alone are contraindicated as they may leave the α-adrenoreceptor–mediated effects of the disorder unopposed. Clonidine is a useful test for the disorder; peripheral catecholamine levels will not be depressed after patients with pheochromocytoma take clonidine, whereas normal subjects will show a prompt decline. Methyldopa is likely to be converted in significant amounts to the weak vasoconstrictor alpha methyl norepinephrine, which may exacerbate the symptoms.

177. The answer is B. *(Organophosphate exposure)*
Organophosphates are highly toxic insecticides that occasionally affect agricultural workers. They are also frequently the primary agent in chemical weapons. They are highly lipid-soluble and are absorbed through virtually all body parts, including the skin. They produce a cholinergic crisis secondary to inhibition of acetylcholinesterase, whichinvolves nicotinic and muscarinic receptors, both centrally and systemically. Atropine decreases some ofthe muscarine effects, including the bronchospasm and increased secretions of the airways. Mechanical ventilation may still be required if respiratory muscles are paralyzed. Pralidoxime, if given early enough, will help regenerate new cholinesterase and ultimately hasten reversal of the overdose.

178. The answer is C. *(Self-tolerance)*
The thymus is an antigenically privileged site, and thymocytes pass through only once; therefore, peripheral tolerance may be a necessary mechanism. There is no evidence that T cells leave and then come back to the thymus. Tolerance seems to be a negative-selection phenomenon, and it is believed that all selection initially takes place in the thymus.

179–183. The answers are: 179-D, 180-B, 181-C, 182-C, 183-B. *(Embryology)*
Ectoderm gives rise to the nervous system, sensory epithelia, epidermis, mammary glands, and the pituitary gland. Melanocytes in the dermis arise from neuroectoderm. Mesoderm gives rise to cartilage, bone, connective tissue, muscles, the cardiovascular system, kidneys, gonads, spleen, and the adrenal cortex. Endoderm gives rise to gastrointestinal and respiratory mucosa, and the parenchyma of the tonsils, thyroid gland, parathyroid glands, thymus, liver, and pancreas.

184–186. The answers are: 184-C, 185-A, 186-B. *(Hepatic histology)*
This is a scanning electron micrograph of the liver. Liver parenchymal cells (*A*) secrete bile into the bile canaliculi (*B*) and blood proteins, such as serum albumin and transferrin, into the liver sinusoids (*C*).

Liver sinusoids are modified fenestrated and discontinuous capillaries that receive blood from the portal vein and hepatic artery in the portal canals and carry it to the central veins.

187–191. The answers are: 187-E, 188-D, 189-C, 190-B, 191-A. *(Lipoproteins and genetic disorders)*
Lipoprotein lipase is an enzyme normally located within the capillary endothelium; it is involved in converting chylomicrons to chylomicron remnants. A deficiency in lipoprotein lipase leads to elevated circulating levels of chylomicrons. Chylomicron levels may also be elevated in systemic lupus erythematosus (SLE).

Familial hypercholesterolemia, due to mutation within a single gene, is one of the most common human mendelian disorders. Low-density lipoprotein (LDL) levels are elevated in the serum because this disorder markedly decreases the number of high-affinity LDL receptors within the liver. LDL levels may also be elevated in nephrotic syndrome and hyperthyroidism.

Familial (type III) hyperlipoproteinemia has been traced to a single amino acid substitution within the receptor for apoprotein E. As the apoprotein E receptor is required for the normal metabolism of both chylomicron remnants and intermediate-density lipoproteins (IDL), both of these molecules accumulate in the blood.

The biochemical defect underlying familial hypertriglyceridemia is unknown. In this disorder, serum levels of both very low-density lipoprotein (VLDL) and triglycerides are elevated. VLDL and triglyceride levels may also be elevated in diabetes mellitus and chronic alcoholism.

The defect underlying familial hyperlipidemia is unknown, although research suggests a deficiency in apoprotein CII. In this disorder, serum levels of VLDL and chylomicrons are elevated; alcoholism, diabetes mellitus, and oral contraceptives are also capable of elevating VLDL and chylomicron levels.

192–196. The answers are: 192-B, 193-C, 194-A, 195-D, 196-E. *(Neuroanatomy)*
Many neuroanatomic pathways now can be specified by their neurotransmitters. Thus, selective depletion of the neurotransmitters can be caused by sectioning of pathways or by destroying the perikarya that produce the neurotransmitter.

Destruction of interneurons of the spinal cord would deplete γ-aminobutyric acid (GABA) and glycine, inhibitory transmitters produced by interneurons. Dorsal root section would reduce substance P concentration in the dorsal horns. This neurotransmitter presumably transmits pain impulses from the small fibers in the lateral division of the dorsal roots. Destruction of the substantia nigra would deplete dopamine, the major neurotransmitter within the basal ganglia. Section of the medial forebrain bundle would destroy many of the axons that connect the catecholaminergic and serotoninergic nuclei of the brain stem with the cerebral cortex. Destruction of the medullary raphe would destroy the serotoninergic neurons of the medulla that project to the spinal cord.

Not only can the neurotransmitters be depleted by actual anatomic destruction of axonal pathways or the destruction of neuronal perikarya, but various drugs and chemicals can also selectively block neurotransmitters either by inhibiting their formation, inhibiting their release, or competing with binding sites on the postsynaptic membrane. By combining anatomic lesions with chemical blockade and direct chemical analysis, various lines of evidence can be developed to establish the transmitters involved in the various layers and regions of the cortex and the different nuclei of the central nervous system (CNS).

197–200. The answers are: 197-A, 198-C, 199-B, 200-E. *(Oncogenes; oncogenesis; signal transduction; growth factor receptors)*
Alteration of virtually any cellular signaling system has the potential for causing oncogenesis. The *ros* oncogene product is an activated insulin receptor. The homolog of one of the two subunits of the nerve growth factor (NGF) receptor is *trk*. The oncogene *erbB* has activated tyrosine kinase, which is also activated when epidermal growth factor (EGF) binds to the EGF receptor. The oncogenic homolog of the platelet-derived growth factor (PDGF) receptor is *kit*, while *sis* binds to the PDGF receptor. The nuclear oncogene *jun* is involved in the control of gene transcription.

201–206. The answers are: 201-E, 202-A, 203-C, 204-A, 205-D, 206-B. *(Etiology of spirochetal diseases)*
Borrelia recurrentis is the etiologic agent of relapsing fever in humans. The disease occurs worldwide and is characterized by a febrile bacteremia. The disease name is derived from the fact that 3–10 recurrences can occur, apparently from the original infection. The disease is transmitted to humans from infected animals by ticks and from human to human by lice.

Bejel is nonvenereal, endemic syphilis caused by a variant of *Treponema pallidum*. The disease usually is seen in children in the Middle East and Africa. Transmission appears to be through the shared use of drinking and eating utensils; bejel is not transmitted sexually. The disease develops in primary, secondary, and tertiary stages.

Pinta is a tropical disease caused by *Treponema carateum*. It occurs primarily in Central and South America, where it appears to be spread by person-to-person contact. Unlike other treponemal diseases, the lesions of pinta remain localized in the skin.

The etiologic agent of syphilis is *T. pallidum*. Humans are the only natural host of the spirochete, and venereal transmission is the most common means of acquiring the infection. Congenital syphilis occurs when the fetus is infected transplacentally and survives to delivery. Accidental laboratory infections occasionally occur.

Fort Bragg fever is a localized name of pretibial fever caused by *Leptospira interrogans* serogroup *autumnalis*. The disease is characterized by a rash on the shins. Humans probably acquire the infection by contact with the urine of infected animals.

Treponema pertenue is the etiologic agent of yaws. The disease occurs primarily in children in tropical regions, where it appears to be transmitted by direct contact or by vectors such as flies. This potentially disfiguring disease has primary, secondary, and tertiary stages.

207–212. The answers are: 207-A, 208-C, 209-B, 210-B, 211-A, 212-A. *(Abnormal heart sounds)*
The first heart sound, S_1, is composed of the sounds of tricuspid and mitral valve closure. Mitral valve closure is normally almost silent, and S_1 is normally quieter than the second heart sound, S_2, which is the sound of the aortic and pulmonic valves closing. S_1 is better heard at the apex of the heart, and S_2 is better heard at the base of the heart. With mitral valve stenosis, the left ventricle is underfilled at the end of diastole, and its systolic contraction has force sufficient to cause the mitral valve leaflets to close audibly. During ventricular systole, the presence of aortic stenosis produces a high flow rate through the stenotic valve, which is appreciated as a pansystolic murmur. The sound is heard well at both the base and apex of the heart and is relatively unchanged by respiratory movements. In acute aortic regurgitation, the left ventricle is overfilled, and the ejection fraction is reduced. During ventricular systole, the pressure buildup is more sluggish than normal due to the leaking aortic valve. The mitral valve closure becomes even quieter than normal; thus, S_1 is quieter than normal. In systemic hypertension, the higher than normal pressure within the aortic bulb at the end of systole causes the very forceful closure of the aortic valve, which produces an S_2 that is louder than usual. In cases of severe anemia or hyperthyroidism, the heart rate is increased along with cardiac output. The increase in heart rate causes the heart to spend a greater portion of its time in systole and less time in diastole. The reduction in diastolic time means that the left ventricle may be relatively underfilled at the beginning of systole. As stated above, the contraction of an underfilled ventricle allows the mitral valve to close with force sufficient to cause S_1 to be louder than S_2.

213–216. The answers are 213-C, 214-D, 215-A, 216-B. *(Degenerative joint disease)*
Rheumatoid arthritis is a common chronic inflammatory disease affecting the joints. Initially the small joints of the hands and feet are involved. The disease is strongly associated with genetic factors — over 75% of Caucasians affected have human leukocyte antigen DR4 (HLA-DR4).

Osteoarthritis is characterized by progressive deterioration of the articular cartilage of weight-bearing joints. Erosion of cartilage eventually leads to thickening of the underlying bone and to knobby protruding of the bone. These protrusions are called Heberden's nodes. They may break off the bone surface and form intra-articular bodies called "joint mice."

Lyme disease (Lyme arthritis) is caused by *Borrelia burgdorferi*, which is transmitted by ticks, whose reservoirs are field mice and deer. The disease has a spectrum of symptoms similar to those of rheumatoid arthritis, principally affecting the knees. Symptoms may last for a long period of time (months) and may lead to a chronic insidious polyarthritis.

Gout is manifested by hyperuricemia, arthritis (gouty arthritis), and the deposit of tophi (urate crystals) in and around the joints. The tophi are surrounded by histiocytes, giant cells, and fibroblasts, causing inflammation.

217–219. The answers are: 217-F, 218-C, 219-D. *(Valsalva maneuver)*
The subject described in the question exhaled against a small leak, requiring the use of thoracic and abdominal muscles to maintain voluntarily an elevated esophageal (and intrathoracic) pressure of 40 cm H_2O. Transmission of applied pressure causes a rise in blood pressure *(B)* followed quickly by a decrease in arterial pressure and pulse pressure *(C)* as venous return is cut off. A reflex change during the maneuver prevents further decline in blood pressure with accompanying reflex tachycardia *(D)*. When the strain ends, the blood pressure falls, and venous return is restored *(E)*. In a normal subject, an overshoot in pressure followed by a vagally mediated bradycardia ensues *(F)*.

220–224. The answers are: 220-E, 221-A, 222-D, 223-B, 224-A. *(Personality disorders)*
Antisocial behavior as an adult has roots in similar behavior as a child or teenager; such children are termed conduct-disordered. Obsessive–compulsive individuals are overly rigid, perfectionistic, overly organized, and have difficulty relaxing or having fun. Narcissistic individuals are self-centered with a grandiose sense of self, yet they have underlying poor self-esteem and become enraged when they perceive criticism, even if slight. Individuals with borderline personalities frequently cut themselves, even superficially, and often have multiple scars.

225–227. The answers are: 225-B, 226-A, 227-D. *(Inflammatory heart disease)*
Chronic rheumatic heart disease refers to the long-term cardiac complications (especially valvular) of acute rheumatic fever. Typically, the mitral and aortic valve leaflets become thickened and deformed by fibrosis, with commissural fusion. The damaged valves represent a fertile ground for the development of infective endocarditis (subacute type).

Chronic rheumatic heart disease is a complication of acute rheumatic fever, which is a nonsuppurative systemic disorder related to an untreated pharyngitis caused by group A β-hemolytic streptococci. Although the precise mechanism of acute rheumatic fever is unknown, the presence of antistreptococcal antibodies that cross-react with heart antigens in these patients suggests an autoimmune basis for this disorder.

Subacute bacterial endocarditis most commonly is caused by α-hemolytic (viridans) streptococci, organisms that are a normal component of the oral flora. Typically, the organism gains entry to the circulation with minor oral trauma, and a transient bacteremia ensues. The bacteria then colonize a platelet-fibrin thrombus that has formed on a valve previously damaged by chronic rheumatic heart disease, mitral valve prolapse, previous cardiac surgery, or some other cause.

The acute form of bacterial endocarditis, in contrast to the subacute form, typically involves a normal heart valve in the setting of a well-defined bacteremia. In this case, the infectious agent usually is a virulent organism (e.g., *Staphylococcus aureus*) that causes the initial damage to the valves by way of a toxin.

Libman-Sacks endocarditis (also known as nonbacterial verrucous endocarditis) may occur as a complication of systemic lupus erythematosus (SLE). This disorder is characterized by the presence of warty endocardial vegetations along the valve margins and, most distinctively, on the undersurface of the valves.

228–232. The answers are: 228-F, 229-D, 230-A, 231-E, 232-C. *(Tumors of the musculoskeletal system)*
A chondroblastoma is a benign tumor composed of small immature chondrocytes, each with a single nucleus, dispersed among benign-appearing, multinucleated giant cells and chondroid matrix. This tumor most often occurs within the epiphyseal region of long, tubular bones of individuals between the ages of 10 and 20 years. Males are affected twice as often as females.

A giant cell tumor is a benign, but locally invasive, lesion characterized by many multinucleated giant cells distributed in a stroma of neoplastic, smaller, mononucleated cells. Over 50% of these "brown" tumors develop in the distal femur or proximal tibia or fibula. The majority of individuals with this tumor are between 20 and 40 years of age. Females are affected slightly more often than males. The tumor frequently recurs many years after surgical removal.

An osteosarcoma is a malignant tumor that most often arises in the medullary cavity of the metaphyseal end of the long bones of the extremities. It is a tumor of mesenchymal cells in which there is deposition of osteoid or new bone. This tumor is most often seen in adolescent or young adult males. Deletions of the long arm of chromosome 13, which are associated with retinoblastoma, are hypothesized to be associated with osteosarcoma development. Radiographs of osteosarcomas often visualize Codman's triangle — an angle formed between the elevated periosteum and the plane of the outer surface of the cortical bone.

Osteoid osteoma is a small, extremely painful benign tumor without the potential for malignant transformation. Radiographically, it appears as small, radiolucent foci surrounded by dense sclerotic bone. Most lesions are intracortical and arise near the ends of the femur or tibia. The lesion appears most often in individuals between 5 and 25 years of age, and it occurs twice as often in males as in females.

Ewing's sarcoma is a malignant neoplasm, most often seen in the pelvis and long tubular bones. It is characterized radiographically by "onion-skin" layering of the cortex and widening of the diaphyseal region. Ewing's sarcoma usually arises before the age of 20 years, and it appears twice as often in males as in females. This tumor is associated with translocation of portions of the long arms of chromosomes 11 and 22.

The majority of chondrosarcomas affect the pelvis and ribs; they most often occur between the middle and the end of the life span.

233–235. The answers are: 233-C, 234-B, 235-B. *(Anatomy of abdominal fascia)*
The abdominal superficial fascia (subcutaneous tissue) has two layers: The superficial fatty layer is called Camper's fascia; the deep membranous layer is called Scarpa's fascia. Both are especially prominent over the abdominal wall. Of these two layers, only Scarpa's fascia can support sutures. Scarpa's fascia continues over the pubis and perineum as Colles' fascia.

236–243. The answers are: 236-B, 237-B, 238-C, 239-D, 240-A, 241-B, 242-A, 243-B. *(Intestinal diseases)*
Ulcerative colitis usually involves the large intestine, where it commonly causes a diffuse inflammatory reaction that stops abruptly at the terminal ileum. The rectum is invariably involved. The inflammatory reaction involves the mucosa and superficial submucosa and results in crypt abscesses and pseudopolyps. It is associated with a definite increased risk of colonic adenocarcinoma.

Crohn's disease affects the large and small bowel in a segmental fashion, resulting in "skip" lesions. The inflammatory process is transmural, leading to fistulae between adjacent segments of intestine. The characteristic histologic finding is the non-necrotizing granuloma, which may be seen in the inflammatory reaction within the bowel wall or in pericolonic lymph nodes.

244–247. The answers are: 244-A, 245-C, 246-D, 247-C. *(Characteristics of lung carcinomas)*
Oncogene amplification and mutation is in the initial phases of study. However, adenocarcinoma has been shown to have a high incidence of K-*ras* oncogene abnormalities, while small cell carcinoma has an association with c-*myc* gene amplifications. Small cell carcinoma differentiates along neuroendocrine cell lines, which is reflected in the presence of membrane-bound, dense-core neurosecretory granules within the cell cytoplasm. The cytoplasm contains peptide hormones, which induce paraneoplastic syndromes. Bronchioloalveolar adenocarcinoma shares histologic similarity to a virus-induced carcinoma in sheep, called jaagsiekte. Bronchioloalveolar adenocarcinoma is characterized by lepidic growth by mucin-secreting cells and by bronchorrhea.

248–252. The answers are: 248-B, 249-E, 250-A, 251-D, 252-C. *(Neuropathology)*
Neurofibrillary tangles are not unique to Alzheimer's disease as they are also seen in Down syndrome, normal aging, and pugilistic dementia; however, they uniquely occur in high concentrations in the hippocampus of Alzheimer's patients. Multinucleated giant cells occur in patients with AIDS who have encephalitis. Lewy bodies and eosinophilic cytoplasmic inclusions in the substantia nigra, are characteristic of Parkinson's disease. Prions, proteins devoid of nucleic acid that are infectious, are associated with Creutzfeldt-Jakob dementia. Pick's bodies stain silver and are inclusions within neurons.

253–257. The answers are: 253-C, 254-A, 255-B, 256-B, 257-D. *(Neurochemistry)*
Cholinergic neurons of the basal nucleus of Meynert degenerate in Alzheimer's dementia with an associated decrease in choline acetyltransferase. Tyrosine hydroxylase is the rate-limiting step for synthesis of dopamine, norepinephrine, and epinephrine; it forms dopa from tyrosine. The monoamine oxidase (MAO) enzyme for the breakdown of catecholamines and serotonin is located on the mitochondria. Because MAO levels increase with age after 35 years, MAO inhibitors may be particularly useful antidepressant drugs in the elderly. The dorsal raphe nuclei of the pons and medulla constitute an important serotonergic area of the brain. Tryptophan-5-hydroxylase is the rate-limiting enzyme in the synthesis of serotonin.

Whipple's disease is a systemic infectious disorder characterized by periodic acid–Schiff (PAS)-positive macrophages in the lamina propria of the intestines. Significant mucosal and lymphatic destruction lead to clinical manifestations of malabsorption.

Hirschsprung's disease is a congenital defect in which neural crest cells do not undergo their normal caudal migration, effectively denervating the anal sphincter and rectum. Accordingly, the proximal colon becomes dilated.